# The Diagnosis and Treatment of Medicare

AEI STUDIES ON MEDICARE REFORM
Joseph Antos and Robert B. Helms
*Series Editors*

What ails Medicare is what ails health care in America. Medicare spending is growing substantially faster than we can afford, with potentially disastrous consequences for the federal budget. Worse, although the program is paying for more services, it is not necessarily providing better care for the elderly and the disabled. AEI's Studies on Medicare Reform is designed to examine the program's operation, consider alternative policy options, and develop a set of realistic proposals that could form the basis for reform legislation.

THE DIAGNOSIS AND TREATMENT OF MEDICARE
*Andrew J. Rettenmaier and Thomas R. Saving*

# The Diagnosis and Treatment of Medicare

Andrew J. Rettenmaier and
Thomas R. Saving

The AEI Press

*Publisher for the American Enterprise Institute*

WASHINGTON, D.C.

Distributed to the Trade by National Book Network, 15200 NBN Way, Blue Ridge Summit, PA 17214. To order call toll free 1-800-462-6420 or 1-717-794-3800. For all other inquiries please contact the AEI Press, 1150 Seventeenth Street, N.W., Washington, D.C. 20036 or call 1-800-862-5801.

Library of Congress Cataloging-in-Publication Data

Rettenmaier, Andrew J.
  The diagnosis and treatment of medicare / by Andrew J. Rettenmaier and Thomas R. Saving.
      p. cm.
  Includes bibliographical references and index.
  ISBN-13: 978-0-8447-4251-9
  ISBN-10: 0-8447-4251-1
  1. Medicare. 2. Medicare—Finance. 3. Health care reform—United States. I. Saving, Thomas Robert, 1933- II. American Enterprise Institute for Public Policy Research. III. Title.
  [DNLM: 1. Medicare—economics. 2. Health Care Reform—economics—United States. 3. Medicare—organization & administration. WT 31 R439d 2007]
      RA412.3.R4798 2007
      368.4'2600973—dc22

                                                              2007007413

11 10  09  08  07        1  2  3  4  5

*Printed in the United States of America*

# Contents

# List of Illustrations

TABLES

# Acknowledgments

The authors express their sincere appreciation to the Lynde and Harry Bradley Foundation and the National Center for Policy Analysis for their financial support of the research underlying this work. The authors thank everyone at the AEI Press for their excellent work on this project. In particular, we thank Samuel Thernstrom for keeping the project on schedule and for coordinating each stage of production, and Lisa Ferraro Parmelee for her great attention to detail, her many helpful suggestions, and for all of the extra hours she devoted to the book so it could be finished in a timely manner. We would also like to Barbara Fisher, Amy Hopson, and Missy King for editing early drafts of the chapters.

# 1

# The Medicare Problem and Its Potential Solution

This book is about rethinking Medicare's financing, its benefit structure, and its future. Before such rethinking can be done, a thorough understanding of the health of the program is necessary—hence, the title of this work. To treat the problems of Medicare, we must diagnose its true malady.

Here we do the equivalent of an MRI on Medicare. Looking at its inner workings, we can see clearly the nature and extent of its ailments and then analyze the efficacy of various treatment regimens that have been proposed. In the end, our goal is to contribute to the debate that must soon begin if we are to deal with Medicare's rapidly deteriorating financial condition.

Throughout the discussion, we will be reminded of Medicare's rising cost. Indeed, across the ideological spectrum there is agreement that it will soon surpass Social Security as the largest federal entitlement program, and that together the two programs will dominate the federal budget within a few decades. By 2028, total Medicare spending will exceed total Social Security spending; in 2033, claims on the economy imposed by the two programs combined will rival the size of the rest of today's federal budget as a share of the nation's gross domestic product (GDP).

In Medicare's case, the spending growth is fueled, on the one hand, by demographic forces, and, on the other, by growth in per-capita health-care spending in excess of per-capita GDP growth. The demographic forces are a combination of the retirement of the baby boom generation, improvements in mortality rates, and a drop in fertility. The growth of per-capita health-care expenditures is the result of improvements in technology and the effect of increasing per-capita income on the demand for health care.

As the leading edge of the baby boom generation reaches Medicare eligibility age in 2011, we will see the beginning of a rapid deterioration in the program's finances. By 2030, one year after the last of the baby boomers become eligible for benefits, Medicare spending by itself is projected to account for 6.5 percent of GDP. In addition to this rapid rise in the number of beneficiaries, inflation-adjusted per-capita Medicare spending will increase from $10,685 in 2006 to $18,116 in 2030, for a real annual growth rate of 2.2 percent, according to projections from the Medicare Board of Trustees.[1] In contrast, per-capita real GDP is projected to grow at an annual rate of only 1.1 percent. With its growth rate exceeding that of the economy, average Medicare spending will increase from an amount equal to 23 percent of per-capita income today to more than 30 percent by 2030.

While there is agreement that Medicare and Social Security will grow significantly, there is substantial disagreement as to how their increased claims on the federal budget should be handled. Medicare spending is rising, but its dedicated revenues from payroll taxes and premium payments are not increasing rapidly enough to forestall the need for greater federal contributions to the program. To meet the future revenue requirements, taxes will have to be raised, other federal programs will have to be cut, or retirees will have to pick up more of the tab for their own health-care consumption.

Given the general consensus that Medicare's financial future is bleak, the large number of proposals for reform is not surprising. In evaluating any particular proposal, we must ask two basic questions: First, does the reform curb growth in per-capita costs without sacrificing the quality of care? Second, will future taxpayers foot the bill, or will future retirees have to pay some or all of the expected costs of the reform? Or, put another way, which generation will pay for the rising cost of elderly entitlements?

The ominous projections from the trustees should make future taxpayers wary regarding the future of the Medicare program. However, most future taxpayers are either yet to be born or too young to vote. While the

---

1. Throughout this book we will rely on the projections made by the trustees of the Medicare Trust Fund in the *2006 Annual Report of the Boards of Trustees of the Federal Hospital Insurance and Federal Supplementary Medical Insurance Trust Funds* (U.S. Department of Health and Human Services 2006), hereafter the *2006 Medicare Trustees Report*. In particular, in that report the trustees projected 2006 per-capita Medicare expenditures at $10,685.

projections imply a dramatic increase in the Medicare tax burden, they are made with the assumption that the program will continue in its current form. If fundamental health-care reform were to make consumers more aware of the cost of care, then the level of per-capita health-care expenditures would fall, and perhaps the growth rate in those expenditures would fall as well.

## Medicare in the Context of the American Health-Care Market

The growth in national health-care spending since 1960 and the composition of that spending by the source of funding are illustrated in figure 1-1. In 2004, spending on health-care services and supplies accounted for about 15 percent of GDP, up from 4.7 percent in 1960. Each payment source, with the exception of consumer out-of-pocket payments, had grown as a share of GDP. For example, private insurance payments for health services and supplies grew from 1.1 percent to 5.6 percent of GDP, while federal payments grew from only 0.4 percent to 4.8 percent, between 1960 and 2004. In contrast, consumer out-of-pocket payments for health-care services and

FIGURE 1-1

COMPOSITION OF SPENDING ON HEALTH-CARE SERVICES AND
SUPPLIES AS A PERCENTAGE OF GDP

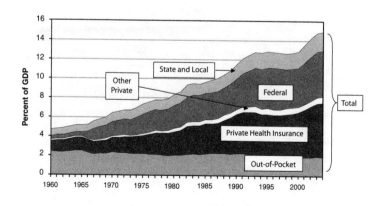

SOURCE: National Health Expenditures 1960–2004.

supplies actually declined, from 2.45 percent of GDP in 1960 to 2.01 percent in 2004.

Figure 1-2 illustrates the changing payment patterns in another way. Here, the total spending in each year is allocated to the various payment sources. The federal government's share has grown the most dramatically, rising from 8.6 percent of spending in 1960 to 32 percent in 2004. While the passage of the legislation establishing Medicare and Medicaid in 1965 has little or no discernable effect on the growth rate of health care as shown in figure 1-1, its effect on who pays for health care is clearly evident.

In 1965, the federal government's share of spending on health-care services and supplies was 8.4 percent, and by 1967, it had risen to 21.7 percent. Private insurance accounted for 23.5 percent of the total in 1960 and 37.7 percent by 2004. State and local government spending as a share of the total was relatively constant. The most striking change in payment patterns occurred in out-of-pocket payments. Individuals paid for 52 percent of their health care in 1960 but only 13.4 percent by 2004. Thus, all of the growth in health-care spending as a share of GDP was paid for by third parties.

FIGURE 1-2

COMPOSITION OF SPENDING ON HEALTH-CARE SERVICES AND
SUPPLIES AS A PERCENTAGE OF THE TOTAL

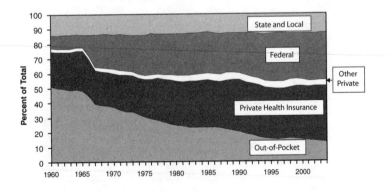

SOURCE: National Health Expenditures 1960–2004.

## Does Who Pays for Health-Care Expenditures Matter?

The prominence of third-party payers in the health-care industry has affected at least the level of expenditures and perhaps even the growth rate in these expenditures. To get a feel for the impact of third-party payments and the rise in real per-capita spending, we present in table 1-1 the average level of third-party payments by health-care sector for the period 1960–85, along with the change in real per-capita spending.

TABLE 1-1
WHO PAYS FOR REAL SPENDING GROWTH? 1960–85

| Spending Category | Percent Paid by Consumers | Percent Real Per-Capita Spending Growth |
|---|---|---|
| Hospital Care | 10.5 | 286 |
| Physician Services | 42.8 | 259 |
| Dental Services | 82.5 | 136 |
| Prescription Drugs | 79.9 | 74 |

SOURCE: National Health Expenditures 1960–2004.

The table clearly shows for this time-span a strong relationship between how much consumers paid and the rate at which the cost of the relevant category rose. Health insurance began as hospital insurance, and the share of hospital care paid for directly by consumers has been low for at least fifty years. For the period in question, consumers paid, on the average, only 10.5 percent of the cost of hospital care, while real per-capita spending rose by 286 percent (5.6 percent annually). Consumers paid for 42.8 percent of their consumption of physician services while real per-capita spending rose 259 percent (5.3 percent annually). In two areas where third-party participation is fairly recent, dental services and prescription drugs, real per-capita expenditure growth was much lower, with a rise of 136 percent for dental services and only 74 percent for prescription drugs (respectively, 3.5 and 2.3 percent annually).

Two issues arise in using this information to infer any form of causality. First, the time period summarized in the table ended twenty years ago.

Second, pharmaceuticals have experienced the highest rate of real cost inflation in recent years. On the first point, we used the 1960–85 data because third-party payments were relatively stable within categories for those years. On the second, disentangling the causality of the change in third-party payments and the rise in expenditures is difficult. We present evidence of this rise and its relationship to per-capita growth in pharmaceutical expenditures in figure 1-3. The evidence here is clearly consistent with the hypothesis that the level of health-care expenditures has been influenced by the third-party system.

FIGURE 1-3

PER-CAPITA PRESCRIPTION DRUG EXPENDITURES AND
THE SHARE PAID BY THIRD PARTIES

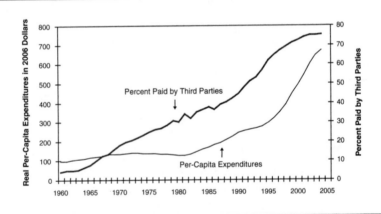

SOURCE: National Health Expenditures 1960–2004.

## A Brief History of Medicare's Costs

Medicare mirrors the rest of health care in its high annual growth rate over the past forty years. Since its inception, the program has grown from a minuscule share of the nation's output to taking more than 2.5 percent of GDP, projected by the trustees to reach 11 percent by 2080. The past rapid growth in cost is the result of two factors.

First, the absolute number of Medicare enrollees has grown. General population growth increases the number of individuals of all ages in the population without changing the distribution across age. However, the forty years of the Medicare program have seen significant improvements in mortality rates, resulting in a growing share of the population that is aged. These improvements in mortality have resulted in the program's participants remaining in it longer and thus contributing to the increase in the absolute size of the Medicare population. In figure 1-4, we show the number of enrollees from the inception of the program through 2005 for the two parts of Medicare in the original legislation.

Medicare Part A, Hospital Insurance, is the mandatory part of the program, in which everyone with a work history of forty quarters in covered employment is enrolled. Medicare Part B, Supplemental Medical Insurance, is a voluntary program that requires participants to pay a premium. However, the Part B premium has always been heavily subsidized. When the program began, the premiums were set at 50 percent of per-capita cost. The subsidy was gradually increased until, by 1980, premiums were set at their current level of 25 percent of per-capita costs. As a result, the Part B enrollment has always been about 95 percent of those eligible to participate.

FIGURE 1-4

**MEDICARE ENROLLMENT TRENDS, 1966–2005**

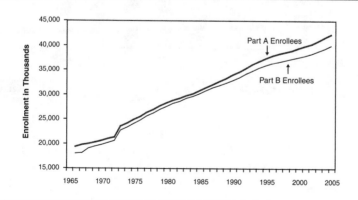

SOURCE: National Medicare Enrollment Trends, CMS website http://www.cms.hhs.gov/MedicareEnrpts/.

From figure 1-4, it is apparent that enrollment has increased steadily from the inception of Medicare to the present. The jump in 1972 was the result of the inclusion of the disabled in the eligible population. Over the entire period, the number of enrollees more than doubled, from 19 million in 1966 to 42 million in 2005. However, this doubling in enrollment was accompanied by a more than tenfold increase in the total cost of Medicare adjusted for inflation. Figure 1-5 shows the level of real per-beneficiary benefits for each five-year period from 1970 to 2005. Expressing everything in 2006 dollars, we find total real per-beneficiary cost rose from $1,793 in 1970 to $8,285 in 2006. The figure also clearly illustrates the increasing role played by Medicare Part B, whose per-capita cost rose much faster than that of Part A.

FIGURE 1-5
REAL AVERAGE MEDICARE COSTS PER BENEFICIARY

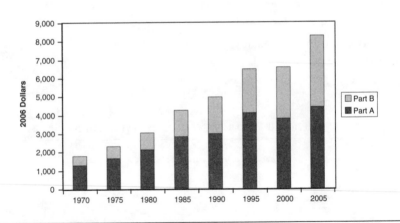

SOURCE: Table V. B1, 2006 Medicare Trustees Report. CPI-W used to adjust past costs for inflation.

Given the rapid increase in the per-beneficiary cost and the doubling of the Medicare population, it is not surprising that the total cost of the program has become an increasing share of the nation's GDP. Figure 1-6 depicts the path of total Medicare spending and Medicare spending net of the premiums paid by participants and demonstrates the rapid growth of the program as a share of GDP.[2] When Medicare began, its cost was a minimal part of GDP—less than two-tenths of 1 percent. By the close of the period, it exceeded 2.5 percent.

FIGURE 1-6

MEDICARE SPENDING AS A PERCENTAGE OF GDP
FROM THE PROGRAM'S INCEPTION UNTIL 2005

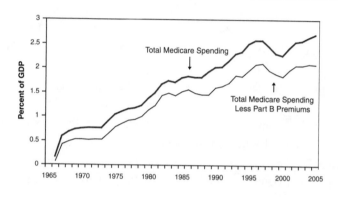

SOURCES: Authors' estimates based on Tables 8.A1 and 8.A2, *Annual Statistical Supplement to the Social Security Bulletin, 2005* and *2006 Social Security Trustees Report* and *2006 Medicare Trustees Report.*

### Some General Issues

For the past fifty years, federal spending, including entitlement spending, has averaged 20 percent of GDP. Assuming Medicare and Social Security grow as projected by the trustees, and all other government programs remain at their current shares of GDP, total federal spending will rise from its 2004 level of 19.5 percent to 25.4 percent of GDP over the next twenty-five years, and to 28.2 percent over the next fifty years. These increases represent, respectively, 30 percent and 44 percent increases in the federal government's share of the economy. Retirees are scheduled to pay for some of this projected growth through their premium payments and general

---

2. Participation in Part B requires a premium, as we have noted above. However, individuals who are not eligible for Part A can choose to participate by paying a premium.

taxes, but most of the increasing cost of government will be borne by future taxpayers.[3]

Some observers point out that the projected federal government share of the economy implied by the growth of these elderly entitlement programs is somewhat comparable to government shares already existing in other developed countries. One could even go as far as to suggest that because other developed countries have government sectors already as big as that predicted for the United States, we need not worry. While the government sector for the United States may be small by international standards, however, allowing it to grow as a share of the economy simply passes the buck to yet-to-be-born citizens and ignores the fundamental issue of generational equity.

This most basic of the issues must be addressed in reforming elderly entitlements, but several other questions arise as well when one tries to tackle the issues related to financing Medicare's projected growth. Primary among these is, are health-care services special? Government policy surely treats them so. Federal and state and local governments pay for 45 percent of national health expenditures. On top of that, health insurance paid for through employers is afforded preferential tax treatment. Compensation in the form of health insurance is not taxable for employees and, as a result, payroll and federal and state income taxes are avoided. This represents a subsidy in the purchase of health insurance.

Employer-provided health insurance became more common during World War II, when wage and price controls prevented firms from raising wages in response to increased demand for labor. Fringe benefits, including health insurance, were not subject to these wartime controls, which prompted firms to add them to their compensation packages as a means to recruit and retain workers. The newly added health-insurance benefits attained favorable status as nontaxable income, based on a 1943 ruling by the Internal Revenue Service.

Currently, over 70 percent of Americans with health insurance of any type, public or private, are covered by a group health plan provided through an employment relationship. It has been estimated that this

---

3. In 1998, income tax revenues from taxpayers ages sixty-five and over accounted for only 2.7 percent of all federal personal income tax revenues.

subsidy results in an annual loss of $188.5 billion in federal tax revenues (Sheils and Haught 2004). The favorable tax treatment results in a lower relative price of health insurance and is responsible, in some part, for the growth in health-care spending. It is likely also a contributing factor in the relatively faster growth in per-capita health-care spending. A leading health economics textbook argues that without the tax subsidy for health insurance, "the health sector would be at least 10 to 20 percent smaller," which translates into "1.5 to 3.0 percent of the gross national product" (Phelps 1997, 357).

Government provision, purchase subsidies, and preferential tax treatment are often advocated if private-market outcomes result in underprovision of a good or service. Underprovision can arise if the good or service in question has the characteristics of a public good, or its consumption produces external costs or benefits. We can ask if health care falls into one of these categories and, if so, whether the current degree of government intervention is justified. Particular areas of health-care spending might be considered public goods—basic research, for example, where it might be argued that since the full returns cannot be captured by those engaging in the research, they cannot all be internalized. Individual spending on the prevention of communicable diseases and health benefits for low-income families also produces returns that accrue to others and will not be internalized by investors. Aside from areas like these, however, most health-care expenditures directly benefit the individual consumer without producing external benefits. How much of this spending is of the pure public-good nature is debatable, but it would be difficult to argue that the current level of government provision, combined with the tax subsidy, is justified.

Another issue that must be addressed in our discussion of Medicare's future is whether health care must be delivered equitably within a generation. For much of the previous century, the goal of equal access to health care was pursued by many politicians and policymakers. Included in Franklin D. Roosevelt's economic bill of rights was "the right to adequate medical care and the opportunity to achieve and enjoy good health."[4] We will discuss social insurance in greater depth in a later chapter, but we can note here that the notion of "the right to adequate medical care" has

---

4. Roosevelt 1944.

evolved to imply that individuals are entitled to the same health-care interventions regardless of their ability to pay for them. In the minds of many, equal interventions have come to be synonymous with equal access. This logic of equity within generations drives much of the policy discussion today, from dealing with the uninsured to equity in the delivery of care to the retired Medicare population.

Most health-care spending is associated with unlikely events that are inherently hard to predict and, potentially, extremely expensive to remedy. Illness or injury may also be associated with loss of earnings for a period of time and may affect future earning capabilities. Aware of these conditions, fully informed consumers would purchase insurance to protect against the risks. Left on their own, they would choose different levels of insurance covering differing degrees of interventions, with interventions varying as a result. Risk-averse individuals would buy more insurance, as would those at high risk of health problems. Wealthier individuals would buy more insurance than lower-income individuals, given that they have more assets to lose. The uninsured would be those with a lower subjective probability of illness and those with fewer assets to insure against losses.

The preferential tax treatment afforded to health insurance purchased through employers has led to the overwhelming share of health care being ˙paid by third-party payers. As a result, most health-care consumption choices, both for the working and retired population, are based on a cost to the consumer that bears little or no relationship to the resource cost of the product being consumed. Furthermore, the effect of any single use of the health-care system has little or no effect on the ability of the user to purchase nonhealth goods or services. Thus, during their working years, individuals consume more health care than they would have purchased if each purchase directly affected their other consumption. Then, as individuals move from working to retirement, it may be unreasonable to expect them to reduce, or even require them to pay for, a greater share of their health-care consumption, especially during a phase of life in which they expect increased use of health-care services.

Medicare reform cannot occur in a vacuum. Any attempt to stem the growth in spending must be consistent with reforms that affect younger Americans. The growth in health-care spending as a percentage of the nation's economy is not necessarily a bad thing. Since there is little apparent concern about the share of GDP used up by other components of consumption, why the concern about the share going to health care? The answer is simple: Individuals pay directly for their consumption of nonhealth goods and services, whereas health-care consumption is paid for either directly by the government or through third parties. As a result, something akin to "the tragedy of the commons" occurs, and individuals consume more health care than they would if they were paying for it directly. Put differently, if individuals paid for health care in the same way they pay for other consumer goods, an increase in the consumption of health care would imply an immediate and equal reduction in other consumption. When the health-care consumption decision has an impact on other consumption equal to the full cost of providing the health care, individuals would consume less. While we do not propose to determine what Americans consume or how much they consume, one of our purposes here is to point to various economic distortions that may lead to more or less health-care consumption than is optimal.

## An Overview of the Book

Our primary purpose in this book is to make the problems inherent in Medicare's financial future apparent, in part by seeking to understand its past, and then to evaluate the contributions that suggested solutions to the coming deficits can make in solving the problem. We accomplish this by presenting the financial deficits projected by the Medicare trustees in ways that make their burden understandable and transparent.

Once the extent of the future burden is clear, the question becomes one of finding ways to finance or eliminate it. Since the rapid growth of Medicare has been with us for some time, suggestions for dealing with the issue abound. Surprisingly, very few of them have been put to the ultimate test of measuring the extent to which they actually solve Medicare's future financial problems. Here we do exactly this, measuring for several prominent proposals.

Finally, we outline a proposal to prepay a restructured Medicare insurance package rather than to continue relying on transfers from taxpayers to beneficiaries. Moving to prepayment will address generational equity by tying the quantity of retirement health care directly to its consumers. Given the projected size of the Medicare program, the question of the benefit package that should be prepaid must be answered. Thus, before we get to a specific proposal for prepaying Medicare, we address the components of a reformed Medicare.

We begin in chapter 2 with an overview of the magnitude of the financing problem, based on the projections in the *2006 Medicare Trustees Report* for the current program. Then, in chapter 3, the burden on future taxpayers is estimated, assuming that the projected deficits are realized, and that these deficits are financed through taxation. In chapter 4, the projections are used to estimate Medicare's burden on the elderly if they are required to pay for the funding shortfalls. In chapters 5–8, we evaluate five Medicare reforms and show the degree to which projected deficits are reduced. In chapter 9, we review the five reform outcomes and compare them in terms of their abilities to alleviate the projected funding problems.

Ultimately, we know that the Medicare deficits cannot persist indefinitely, and, in fact, legislation requires that funding deficits in excess of 45 percent of the program's cost be addressed with a solution. Thus, alternatives will be adopted. An important alternative to the current generational-transfer method of financing Medicare is prepayment through some form of cohort-based financing. Chapter 10 discusses the fundamentals of prepaying retirement health insurance, and chapter 11 presents the cost of prepayment, on a cohort-by-cohort basis, for each of the reforms. These chapters are followed in chapter 12 by our estimates of the annual costs of making the transition to prepaid Medicare.

The notion of "social insurance" is essentially the general agreement among members of a generation that when a pitfall occurs to an individual, others will absorb all or some part of the individual's loss. Such insurance works best when the probability of a loss is low and independent across individual participants in the contract. Given this form of social insurance, how much of Medicare should be part of the social contract? These are the questions that we address in chapter 13. Finally, we conclude with general comments and observations in chapter 14.

# 2

# The Current Status and Future
# of Today's Medicare

Medicare is America's second largest entitlement program, behind Social Security. This year, Medicare is expected to account for 14.0 percent of the federal budget and 3.2 percent of the nation's gross domestic product (GDP), and to require general-revenue transfers equal to 12.3 percent of federal income tax receipts. Medicare provides health-care funding for the retired and disabled population, the same population served by Social Security. The 2003 Medicare Modernization Act (MMA) made the program's coverage more comprehensive with the addition of a prescription drug benefit, which has also made it more costly. By 2028, Medicare spending is expected to exceed Social Security spending, and the differential will continue to escalate thereafter. Further, by the end of the seventy-five-year projection period used in their 2006 report, the Medicare trustees project that Medicare alone will account for 11.0 percent of GDP, or roughly 70 percent of total health-care spending today as a share of GDP.

## The Future Cost of Medicare

Before we begin a detailed discussion of the future of Medicare expenditures, let us review the characteristics that will cause the program to become larger than Social Security in just over twenty years, and 40 percent larger by the middle of this century.

While Social Security and Medicare share the same demographics, the similarity ends there. Social Security's revenue and expenses, without consideration of coming demographic issues, rise at roughly the same pace as the nation's GDP. Thus, its future deficits are the result of the baby boom generation's retirement, falling fertility rates, and lengthening life-spans.

While Medicare faces these same issues, its future financial problems are compounded by the fact that the population's demand for health care is growing faster than the nation's GDP. Since 1960, per-capita health-care expenditures have grown three percentage points faster than per-capita GDP. Medicare Part A Hospital Insurance (HI) tax revenues, however, rise only as fast as GDP, so that even in the absence of demographic issues, Part A would face growing deficits in the future.

Other components of the Medicare program face a similar fiscal situation, but for a different reason. Both parts of Medicare's Supplementary Medical Insurance (SMI), comprised of Part B (physician services) and Part D (prescription drugs), are financed primarily through transfers from federal general revenues.[1] Premium payments from participants in Parts B and D provide only 25 percent and 23 percent, respectively, of program expenditures. General-revenue transfers provide the remaining expenditures— almost 75 percent. Since the premium payments are expected to remain at about their current levels, they will grow as fast as expenditures and, thus, faster than GDP. However, expenditures supplied by general revenues will also grow faster than GDP, implying that an ever-larger proportion of federal general revenues will be required to fund Medicare Parts B and D.

On the revenue side, Part A revenue from HI taxes paid by workers is proportional to GDP growth, and that in the form of premium payments from recipients for Parts B and D is proportional to Parts B and D expenditures. Since taxpayers' share of Medicare revenues is scheduled to grow at the same rate as GDP, and that coming from recipients is scheduled to grow at the same rate as expenditures, recipients will be providing an ever-growing share of total revenues. Premium revenues from Parts B and D beneficiaries, while currently much smaller than HI tax revenues, will ultimately exceed HI tax revenues. In 2005, HI tax revenues were almost

---

1. While we concentrate our analysis on Medicare Parts A, B, and D, there is a Medicare Part C. A combination of A, B, and D, Part C was called Medicare Plus Choice prior to the 2003 Medicare Modernization Act (MMA). It was largely managed care and was declining in importance. After the MMA, Part C became Medicare Advantage, a growing but small part of overall Medicare. Our estimates of overall Medicare that follow include Part C as part of Parts A, B, and D.

five times total Medicare premium income, and in 2007, with the prescription drug benefit fully operational, they will only be 3.5 times premium revenues from beneficiaries. By 2074, Medicare's revenues from premium payments are projected to exceed its revenues from taxation of workers.

In producing the estimates of future Medicare expenditures for their report, the trustees assumed that, by 2030, expenditure growth will have fallen from its current level of approximately 2.0 percentage points faster than per-capita GDP to 1.4 percentage points faster. This slowing was assumed to continue until 2080, when the GDP share of expenditures will stabilize so that the post-2080 growth rate will match that of per-capita GDP.

To see the impact of the historically faster growth of health-care expenditures relative to per-capita GDP growth, we show in figure 2-1 the path of the Medicare expenditures projected by the trustees, and an alternate path whereby per-capita expenditures are restricted to the growth of per-capita GDP. As the figure shows clearly, even when per-capita expenditures are restricted to per-capita GDP growth, the Medicare share of GDP is projected to rise throughout the projection period. This is due to the demographic reality of the retirement of the baby boomers and continuing improvement in longevity. Thus, even if we could stem the historic rapid rise in health-care expenditures, the share of GDP consumed

FIGURE 2-1

**PROJECTED MEDICARE SPENDING IN EXCESS OF GDP GROWTH, 2006–80**

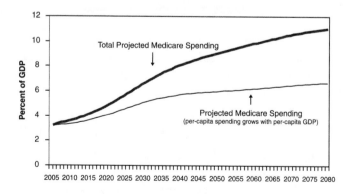

SOURCES: Authors' estimates and Table III.A2., *2006 Medicare Trustees Report*.

by Medicare would rise from its current level of 3.2 percent to 6.7 percent by the close of the trustees' seventy-five-year projection period.

Once we account for the fact that health-care expenditures are growing faster than the economy as a whole and are expected to do so for some time, the growth of Medicare as a share of GDP is even more astounding. The trustees project it will rise from its current level of 3.2 percent to 11.0 percent by 2080. To put this in perspective, note that currently all health care is 16.1 percent of GDP.

Even though the Medicare expenditures projected by the trustees paint a much more daunting picture than that presented by the assumption that per-capita spending grows with per-capita GDP, their prediction that the growth in health-care expenditures will slow to that in per-capita GDP by the close of the seventy-five-year projection period is open to question. While it may be conservative to assume that by 2080 Medicare growth will stabilize at the growth rate of per-capita GDP, there appears to be little evidence that health-care expenditures will not continue to grow faster than per-capita GDP.

### Summary Measures of Medicare's Financial Status

Medicare's financial status can be summarized in two broad ways: first, in terms of the present value of future federal general-revenue requirements, assuming that current-law taxation and premiums remain in effect; and, second, in terms of the path of future budget transfers required to cover the projected funding shortfalls, again assuming that current-law taxation and premiums remain in effect. The first summary measure can be viewed as a representation of the system debt, and the second as the flow of general tax revenue that will be required to meet the projected Medicare obligations. Medicare is fundamentally a generational-transfer system, in that current taxpayers pay for the benefits of current beneficiaries, primarily retirees. If we assume that Medicare will continue as currently structured for the indefinite future, and that the trustees' estimates of that future are valid, then any part of future expenditures that are not covered by dedicated tax and premium revenues must be paid out of other federal revenue sources.

The present value of the flows of resources that will be required to fund Medicare in the future is appropriately viewed as a debt. The trustees calculate this debt in two ways. First, they calculate the present value of the path of resources necessary to cover the projected shortfalls for the seventy-five-year projection period, referred to as the seventy-five-year open-group debt, because as each year passes, new workers enter the labor force and become part of the group being considered. Thus, the open group always consists of all those projected to be living in each of the seventy-five years of the projection. Second, the trustees calculate a closed-group debt, where no new entrants are considered and the revenues projected for only those currently in the system are used to offset the projected benefit costs of those in the system. As each year passes, another birth cohort becomes eligible for Medicare, and eventually all surviving members of the closed group are beneficiaries, but not payroll taxpayers. In general, this second debt, referred to as the hundred-year closed-group debt, is larger than the first because, as the system ages, more and more individuals become beneficiaries, but no new taxpayers enter the system.

Figure 2-2 (on the following page) shows the seventy-five-year unfunded debt based on the *2006 Medicare Trustees Report*. The total unfunded Medicare obligation, defined as projected expenditures in excess of dedicated Medicare taxes and premium payments, is $32.4 trillion.[2] Of this amount, the traditional parts of Medicare, A and B, contribute the lion's share, $24.4 trillion. The newest part of Medicare, the prescription drug benefit, Part D, has a seventy-five-year unfunded general-revenue obligation of $8.0 trillion. We should note here that these figures are based on the liability from the perspective of the Centers for Medicare and Medicaid Services (CMS), and not from the perspective of the federal budget. The CMS treats all revenues, particularly those from premiums, as net revenue. Notably, all premiums for Medicare Parts B and D are treated as net revenue even though some are paid by Medicaid, a program that is jointly funded by federal general revenues and state taxpayers. In contrast, from the perspective of the federal budget, only the premiums actually paid by participants and state taxpayers are, in fact, net

---

2. Thus, the general-revenue transfers that currently finance approximately 75 percent of Parts B and D are included in the definition of unfunded Medicare payments. This approach is appropriate, since these funds are not earmarked for Medicare.

FIGURE 2-2
SEVENTY-FIVE-YEAR UNFUNDED LIABILITY

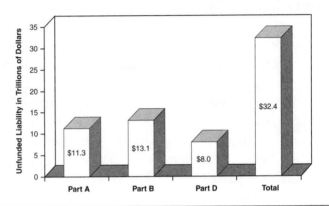

SOURCE: Tables III.B9., III.C15. and III.C21., *2006 Medicare Trustees Report.*

revenue.[3] Further, from the perspective of taxpayers in general, only the premiums paid by participants are net revenue.

It is clear from the magnitude of the seventy-five-year unfunded liability that if these programs remain unchanged, meeting the projected Medicare expenditures, given projected nongovernment revenues, will have a substantial effect on the ability of the federal government to maintain its non-Medicare programs. We address the implications of this more completely in chapter 3.

The seventy-five-year unfunded liability reflects, in a general way, the burden Medicare will place on both current and future generations through the period of the projection. However, two important issues remain. First, what happens after seventy-five years? Do we expect that in that distant future

---

3. This issue became transparent during the 2003 Medicare Modernization Act debate about "dual" eligibles. The total premium income for Part D is projected to be 23 percent of expenditures, but only 12 percent—just over half—will come from beneficiaries who pay their own premiums. The remaining 11 percent will be transferred from the states to the federal government to account for the act's effect on state Medicaid expenditures. Since the states must get the revenue from somewhere, and much of it will come from the federal government, our unfunded liability estimates understate the full liability.

things will level out or just get worse? Second, how is the burden represented in figure 2-2 distributed across current and future generations? Fortunately, the trustees also produce estimates that address the generation-specific burden of future funding shortfalls. If we consider the current generation to be all individuals fifteen years of age and older who are currently alive, then the hundred-year closed-group liability is an estimate of the burden the current generation will impose on those that follow them, assuming the current generation pays only the current-law taxes and premiums and receives the benefits projected by the trustees.[4]

Figure 2-3 shows the debt that will be imposed by the current generation on future ones for each part of Medicare. Those following the current generation—that is, those entering the labor force tomorrow and thereafter—will have to cover this liability under the conditions assumed above. Not surprisingly, the Part A debt is the largest, since its revenues only rise with GDP growth and not with expenditure growth, as they do for Parts B and D.

FIGURE 2-3

**HUNDRED-YEAR CLOSED-GROUP UNFUNDED LIABILITY:
WHAT WE OWE THE CURRENT GENERATION**

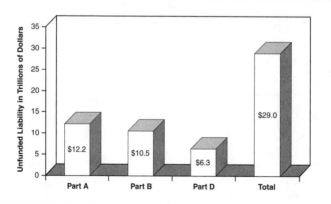

SOURCE: Tables III.B11., III.C16. and III.C22., *2006 Medicare Trustees Report.*

---

4. At the end of one hundred years, the oldest individual in the closed group will be one hundred fifteen years of age. Only one individual in 100,000 will still be alive at that age.

As figure 2-3 shows, the current generation will impose a total debt of $29.0 trillion on future generations. If we give the current generation the projected benefits and only collect the taxes and premiums currently legislated, then subsequent generations will have to cover the entire $29.0 trillion.

The next question is, under current law, how much will these future generations contribute toward the payment of this $29 trillion debt? In figure 2-4, we show the net debt that future generations will impose on the Medicare system, assuming no changes occur in Medicare legislation during the lifetimes of these as-yet unborn generations. Clearly, future generations offer no solution to the financing problem at current tax and premium levels. Rather than providing net revenue to the program, they are projected to impose significant additional costs. For all of Medicare, providing the projected benefits for future generations and only collecting current legislated taxes and premiums implies a net debt for future generations of $41.8 trillion. Thus, if the current level of taxation and premiums continues for the indefinite future, additional federal taxes or a drastically reduced federal government will be required. Again, we will discuss the implications of this in chapter 3.

Combining the data from figures 2-3 and 2-4, we present in figure 2-5 the trustees' estimates of the total debt for each of the three principal programs of Medicare. The total Part A debt is $28.4 trillion, which is the sum

FIGURE 2-4

**DEBT IMPOSED ON THE SYSTEM BY FUTURE GENERATIONS**

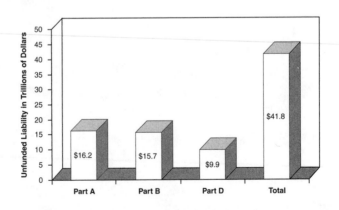

SOURCE: Tables III.B11., III.C16. and III.C22., *2006 Medicare Trustees Report.*

of the $12.2 trillion owed to the current generation and the $16.2 trillion that will be imposed on the system by future generations, due to the excess of their projected benefits over their scheduled tax payments. The total Part B unfunded obligation is $26.2 trillion, the sum of the $10.5 trillion owed the current generation and the $15.7 trillion that will be required to make up the difference between premium income and expenditures for future generations.

Finally, let us consider the newest addition to Medicare, Part D, the prescription drug benefit. Part D is an insurance program in the same sense that Part B is, in that participants are expected to pay premiums that cover only about 23 percent of the total cost.[5] According to figure 2-5, the total Part D unfunded obligation is $16.2 trillion, the sum of the $6.3 trillion owed the current generation and the $9.9 trillion that will be required to make up the difference between premium income and expenditures for future generations.

FIGURE 2-5
TOTAL MEDICARE DEBT

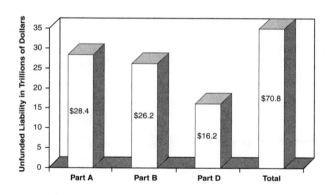

SOURCE: Tables III.B11., III.C16. and III.C22., *2006 Medicare Trustees Report.*

Taking all three parts of Medicare together, the continuation of the current system implies a debt owed to the current generation of $29.0 trillion, and future generations will add another $41.8 trillion to this obligation.

5. This includes premiums paid by Medicaid for eligible Medicare beneficiaries.

Thus, the total Medicare debt is a staggering $70.8 trillion. To put this number in perspective, assume that federal income tax revenues remain at the fifty-year average of 10.8 percent of the nation's gross domestic product for the indefinite future. Under this assumption, the present value of all future federal income tax revenues from now to eternity is $121 trillion, so that the Medicare debt of $70.8 trillion is almost 60 percent of all future federal income tax receipts. If Congress passed legislation today, binding on all future Congresses, that set aside 60 percent of all federal income tax revenues from now to eternity, it would just pay for the promised Medicare benefits. Such a set-aside would imply a substantial reduction in the current role of the federal government.[6]

Another approach to understanding the future funding problems facing Medicare is to review the annual cash flows that will be required if the current system remains in place. These requirements can be denominated in several ways. The first two of these measures—in nominal or in constant dollars—do not contain any frame of reference as to their burden on the economy. Expressing the burden as a share of GDP does give us a frame of reference, but it does not directly bear on the potential burden since no one person owns the GDP—certainly not the government. We prefer to look at the share of projected federal nonentitlement revenues, defined as total federal revenues less revenues earmarked for Social Security and Medicare.

To express the burden Medicare will place on the federal budget in the future, we will compare the required transfers to fund the projected levels of Medicare expenditures as a share of the revenue available to fund federal nonentitlement programs. For example, in 2005, Medicare spending, net of premium payments and dedicated tax revenues, required general-revenue funding equal to 8.1 percent of total nonentitlement revenues.[7]

An 8.1 percent transfer of total nonentitlement revenues may seem like a manageable amount, but two things are worth noting. First, Medicare Part

---

6. Bear in mind that this setting aside of 60 percent of federal income tax revenues cannot be in the form of Treasury bonds sent over to CMS, but must be in the form of real investment in the economy.

7. As a frame of reference, the twenty-five-year average of nonentitlement revenues as a share of GDP is 11.8 percent.

A, the Hospital Insurance portion, went into deficit in 2005 after several years of surplus, and this deficit will grow at an accelerating pace over the next twenty-five years. Second, the budget requirements of Part D, the prescription drug benefit, which began in 2006, will also grow rapidly.

In figure 2-6, we show the transfers required to pay benefits as a share of all federal nonentitlement revenues, given current-law taxes and premiums. These transfers will grow rapidly, from their projected 2006 level of 11.6 percent of the nonentitlement revenues to 21.2 percent in 2020 and to 34.3 percent in 2030, and will require more than two-thirds of all projected nonentitlement revenues by the end of the trustees' seventy-five-year projection period![8]

FIGURE 2-6
**MEDICARE FUNDING SHORTFALLS AS A PERCENTAGE OF
ALL FEDERAL NONENTITLEMENT REVENUES**

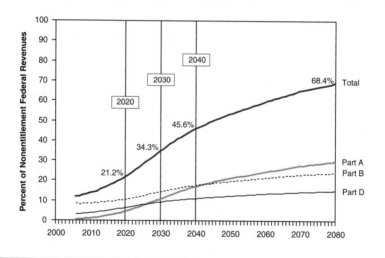

SOURCES: *2006 Medicare Trustees Report* and authors' estimates. Nonentitlement federal revenues estimated to be 11.8 percent of GDP, the 25-year average.

---

8. The projected transfers as a percentage of nonentitlement revenues assume these taxes will equal 11.8 percent of GDP in future years. These percentages can also be thought of as the increase in nonentitlement taxes above their twenty-five-year average share of GDP that would be necessary to meet Medicare's funding requirements.

If the trustees are correct in their projections of Medicare expenditures and the expenditures are unchangeable, the only real alternative to significant increases in taxes on the young is for individual members of society to provide more of the funding for their own retirement health care during their years of work. Alternatively, perhaps regulatory changes to bring about reforms in current Medicare could provide institutions to affect the level of future expenditures without affecting health outcomes. We will address several suggested reforms of Medicare in chapters 5–8.

## Some Further Issues

Two important issues that underlie the projections of the future of Medicare make the projections more uncertain than those for Social Security. First, the trustees assume that certain trends in health-care expenditure growth will ameliorate, but over a very long period of time. Second, they assume that current law remains in place, which, given the provisions of the 2003 MMA, is unlikely to be realized. Each of these issues deserves some attention.

**The Long-Run Growth of Health-Care Expenditures.** Any attempt to make long-run projections of Medicare expenditures requires assumptions concerning the future rate of growth of the health-care sector in general. Specifically, assumptions must be made about the future with reference to GDP that has occurred over the past half-century. Prior to their 2006 report, the trustees assumed the health-care sector would make a gradual transition, over a twenty-five-year period, from its current growth rate of roughly two percentage points faster than per-capita GDP growth to one percentage point faster.[9] This assumption, while perhaps extreme when applied over a seventy-five-year period, results in average growth in health-care expenditures that is well below the rate over the last fifty

---

9. This assumption was put in place in the *2001 Medicare Trustees Report* at the recommendation of the 2000 Medicare Technical Review Panel. The trustees assumed the rate would remain at one percentage point above per-capita GDP growth for the remainder of the seventy-five-year projection period. For projections beyond that time, the trustees assumed that per-capita health-care expenditure growth would equal the growth in per-capita GDP.

years—that is, in the range of two to three percentage points above per-capita GDP growth.

In response to concerns that perpetually faster growth in health-care expenditures would eventually result in all of the nation's output going toward health care, the trustees altered this long-run assumption in their 2006 report. They adopted in its place the assumption that the growth in per-capita health-care costs would slow from its current level of more than two percentage points faster than per-capita GDP to a rate equal to per-capita GDP growth by the close of the seventy-five-year projection period.[10]

While not unreasonable, even this assumption implies that health-care expenditures will rise from today's 16.2 percent of GDP to 32.0 percent by 2040, and that by 2080 they will account for 42.7 percent, with Medicare alone accounting for 11.0 percent. As a result of changing demographics and improving mortality rates, Medicare is projected to grow from its 2006 share of 19.5 percent to 25.7 percent of total health-care expenditures by 2080.

In table 2-1 (on the following page), we show the growth rates of per-capita national health-care expenditures and per-capita GDP for several extended periods. While the growth of health-care expenditures slowed in the 1990s, there is no clear indication of its doing so on a permanent basis. If spending were to rise at a rate equal to per-capita GDP plus one and a half or two percentage points for the entire seventy-five-year projection period, then health care would account for 55 percent or 79 percent of GDP, respectively, by 2075.[11] These implied figures may seem unreasonable, but there are numerous factors contributing to health care growing faster than the rest of consumption.

**Excess General-Revenue Medicare Funding.** Beginning with the *2005 Medicare Trustees Report*, the Medicare Modernization Act required that

---

10. Specifically, the trustees assumed that the per-beneficiary growth rate for all Medicare services would be 1.4 percentage points above GDP growth by 2030. This differential was then assumed to decline gradually to about 0.75 percentage points in 2050 and to less than 0.20 percentage points in 2080. Thereafter, the per-beneficiary growth rate for all Medicare services was assumed to equal GDP growth.

11. Estimates are from *Review of Assumptions and Methods of the Medicare Trustees' Financial Projections*, Technical Review Panel on the Medicare Trustees Reports, December 2000.

TABLE 2-1

REAL PER-CAPITA GROWTH IN NATIONAL HEALTH EXPENDITURES (NHE) VERSUS GROSS DOMESTIC PRODUCT (GDP) IN PERCENT

| Period | NHE | GDP | NHE-GDP |
|---|---|---|---|
| 1945 to 2002 | 4.2% | 1.5% | 2.6% |
| 1960 to 2002 | 4.5 | 1.5 | 3.0 |
| 1970 to 2002 | 4.0 | 1.8 | 2.2 |
| 1980 to 2002 | 4.4 | 2.0 | 2.4 |
| 1990 to 2002 | 3.7 | 1.9 | 1.8 |

SOURCE: *2004 Review of Assumptions and Methods of the Medicare Trustees' Financial Projections.*

the Board of Trustees test whether the difference between program outlays and dedicated financing sources (consisting of HI payroll taxes, the HI share of income taxes on Social Security benefits, Part B beneficiary premiums, and Part D beneficiary premiums plus the state transfers required for dual-eligibles) exceeded 45 percent of total Medicare expenditures. If this critical level were expected to be attained within seven years of the projection for two consecutive years, a determination of "excess general-revenue Medicare funding" would be triggered.

In their 2006 report, the trustees noted that the critical difference would be reached in 2012, within the seven-year requirement, prompting them to issue the determination of "excess general-revenue Medicare funding." If their 2006 forecasts remain on track, a second such determination will be made in the 2007 report, and a "Medicare Funding Warning" will be triggered. This finding will require the president to submit to Congress, within fifteen days after the date of the next budget submission, proposed legislation to respond to the warning. Congress is then required to consider this legislation on an expedited basis.

In figure 2-7, we show the projected path of the general-revenue share of Medicare expenditures based on the 2006 trustees report. According to the trustees' projections, the general-revenue share of total Medicare expenditures will grow rapidly from its current level of 41.3 percent to 53.2 percent in less than fifteen years, and to 62.1 percent by the year 2020; and, by 2040, general revenues will have to supply more than two-thirds of total

Medicare funding. If current law remains in effect, these transfers will place a substantial burden on the remainder of federal government programs. Given the importance of Medicare and the magnitude of the looming deficits, the necessary remedies may be painful.

FIGURE 2-7
**MEDICARE'S GENERAL REVENUE BURDEN**

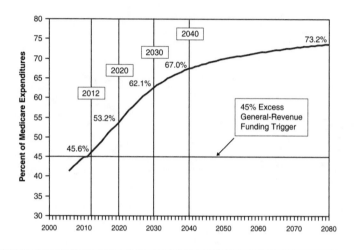

SOURCE: Table III.A2. and Figure III.A1., *2006 Medicare Trustees Report.*

## Conclusion

Medicare's financing problems occur sooner than Social Security's, and their solutions are more difficult. In addition to the general-revenue funding that will be required to cover the deficit in Hospital Insurance (Medicare Part A), Supplementary Medical Insurance (Parts B and D) will require increasing general-revenue transfers with each passing year. The pace of this increase will accelerate as the use of the Part D prescription drug benefit matures. The demands that Medicare, as projected by the trustees, will impose on the rest of the federal budget will force Congress to consider some difficult choices as to who should bear the burden of retirement health-care spending. As the debate over Social Security has highlighted the generational consequences of financing elderly entitlements, the generational burden represented by Medicare amplifies the need for serious consideration of reform. To inform further and form a basis for the subsequent discussion of Medicare reform, the next two chapters present our estimates of the taxes or other means of financing that will be required to fund the level of Medicare expenditures currently projected by the trustees.

# 3

## Paying for Projected Medicare Expenditures: Taxing the Young

Medicare, as it is currently structured, cannot continue. Given the legislative requirements in the Medicare Modernization Act, the implications for government finance imply that significant tax increases or benefit cuts will be required to cover the very significant deficits projected by the Medicare Board of Trustees. To get a feel for the magnitude of the problem, we present here estimates of the revenue that must be raised to cover the projected deficits if no benefit cuts are made. In doing so, we make assumptions concerning the size of other government programs. Our approach, at least initially, will be to assume that the Medicare expenditures projected by the trustees will, in fact, happen. We will also assume that the resources implied by these expenditures will be found, either from additional taxation on workers or additional premiums paid by beneficiaries. In this chapter we address the impact that choosing taxation as the funding source will have on taxpayers and the federal budget.

In the following discussion, Hospital Insurance (Medicare Part A) and Supplemental Medical Insurance (Medicare Part B, outpatient services, and Medicare Part D, prescription drugs) are treated separately, because they are legislatively financed differently. Medicare Part A is financed primarily through the HI payroll tax, currently set at 2.9 percent. Payroll taxes account for about 94 percent of Part A revenues, with almost all of the remainder coming from taxation of Social Security benefits and premiums from voluntary participants in Medicare—that is, those above sixty-five years of age who have not worked forty quarters in covered employment but who choose to take Medicare and pay an actuarially fair premium.[1]

31

### Balancing the Medicare Part A Budget with Payroll Taxation

Since the Part A revenue comes primarily from the payroll tax, it seems natural to begin this discussion by calculating the payroll tax rate that would balance the Part A budget. If we address the future shortfalls through increases in the payroll tax rate, that rate can be expected to rise significantly.

Using the projections underlying the *2006 Medicare Trustees Report* and accounting for both the revenue from premiums and the taxation of Social Security benefits, we show in figure 3-1 the payroll tax rates that will be required to balance the Medicare Part A budget on a continuing basis. From the figure, it is apparent that the payroll tax will immediately begin a slow rise that will accelerate in the middle of the next decade as the front edge of the baby boomers reaches age sixty-five. In 2020, less than fifteen years from now, the HI payroll tax rate will have to rise from its current 2.9 percent level to 4.3 percent. By the year 2030, ten years later, the rate will be 6.0 percent, more than double its current level. By the end of the seventy-five-year projection period, in 2080, it will be 11.6 percent.

Two factors about using payroll taxation to balance the Part A budget make the required rate increases even more worrisome. First, payroll taxes are pre-income-tax dollars. Thus, the tax payments themselves are subject to income taxation. Or alternatively, the money used to pay income taxes is subject to payroll taxation. Clearly, the imposition of two taxes on the same base income has an interaction effect that escalates the government's total take from workers' income. Assuming a 30 percent income tax rate, the projected 2080 11.6 percent Part A payroll tax is the

---

1. The law provides the opportunity to purchase Medicare to individuals sixty-five years of age and over who do not have the required number of quarters to be eligible for the program. Until 1997, the HI premium was based on the overall average cost of providing benefits. Since 1997, the premium has been the 1997 premium adjusted for prices but not expenditures. This is important, because premiums will not rise as fast as the cost of benefits, thus creating another source of future shortfalls. The 1983 Social Security reform provided for the taxation of up to 50 percent of Social Security benefits if recipient income exceeded legislated levels, with the proceeds going to Social Security. In 1992, up to 80 percent of Social Security benefits became subject to income taxation, with the revenues collected from above the 50 percent level dedicated to Medicare Part A. These revenues can be expected to grow as more retirees become subject to Social Security benefit taxation.

FIGURE 3-1

**PAYROLL TAX RATE REQUIRED TO BALANCE THE MEDICARE PART A BUDGET**

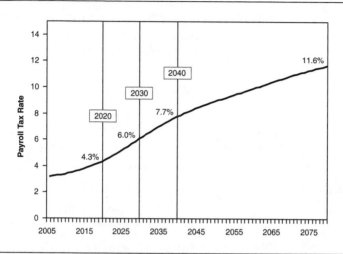

SOURCE: Table VI. F2. *2006 Social Security Trustees Report.*

equivalent of a 15.1 percent tax rate on payroll earnings, or a 33.5 percent tax on funds used to pay income taxes. Second, as we show in the next section, the increase in taxation required to cover the pending deficits—either through increased payroll taxes to cover Part A deficits or increased general income taxation to cover Parts B and D deficits—would constitute a major increase in the overall level of taxation.

## Balancing the Medicare Parts B and D Budgets with General Taxation

When Medicare Part B was established in 1967, the federal government's contribution was set to match the premium contributions of participants, at that time individuals sixty-five years of age and over who were eligible for and participating in Medicare Part A. As a result, 50 percent of Part B costs were to be paid using transfers from federal government general revenues. In 1974, the program was expanded to include eligible disabled individuals under age sixty-five. The newly included disabled were permitted to participate at premium rates that began at roughly 20 percent of total disabled benefits and gradually fell to a low of 13.4 percent in 1984. Beginning in 1976, Part B premiums for participants ages sixty-five and over began a decline, from 50 percent of cost per capita to the current legislated level of 25 percent. For disabled participants in Part B, premiums are currently set at 20 percent of per-capita cost.

In 2005, general-revenue transfers covered 77.7 percent of total Part B expenditures, including the disabled. However, the Medicare Modernization Act of 2003 (MMA) included some means-testing for Part B premiums. MMA means-testing is projected ultimately to reduce the general-revenue share of Part B costs to 74.6 percent from the current long-run legislated level of 75 percent.[2] Because the level of means-testing is so modest, general revenues will continue to provide most Part B revenue requirements. Further, given that total health-care expenditures are rising faster than gross domestic product, the various health-care subsidies will consume a greater and greater share of federal revenues if there are no significant changes in the tax code. For our purposes, we ignore the large role played by the federal government in the health-care industry, concentrating our work on Medicare.[3]

In figure 3-2, we show the projected path of the federal general-revenue transfers required to pay for Medicare Parts B and D, after accounting for premiums paid by participants. We express these transfers as a share of

---

2. The 2003 Medicare Modernization Act introduced a higher "income-related" premium for individuals whose modified adjusted gross income exceeds a specified threshold, set for 2007 at $80,000 for individual returns and $160,000 for joint returns, and then indexed to inflation. Individuals exceeding the threshold will pay premiums covering 35, 50, 65, or 80 percent of average program costs for aged beneficiaries, depending on their income level.

3. We note, however, that the role of the federal government in the provision of health care for the preretirement population, of which Medicaid is an example, coupled with the fact that all health care is growing faster than GDP, implies that the share of federal nonentitlement revenues consumed by health-care provision will rise throughout the period we consider. Thus, holding constant the nonentitlement revenue share of GDP after Medicare transfer will not assure that federal nonhealth expenditures as a share of GDP will remain at current levels. In fact, as federal expenditures on Medicaid rise faster than GDP, non–health-care federal expenditures can be expected to fall even with our restriction of the Medicare transfer.

FIGURE 3-2
MEDICARE PARTS B AND D REQUIRED TRANSFERS

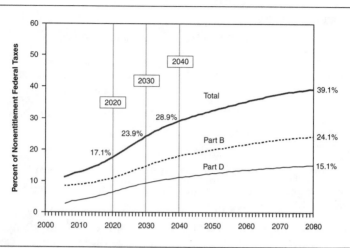

SOURCES: Authors' estimates and *2006 Medicare Trustees Report*.
NOTE: Federal nonentitlement taxes are estimated to be 11.8 percent of GDP, the twenty-five-year average.

federal nonentitlement tax receipts, because these are the only receipts available to fund general expenditures. In 2005, Part B transfers accounted for 7.8 percent of nonentitlement income. This share is rising rapidly, and funding Part B will require 10.7 percent of nonentitlement income by 2020 and 17.7 percent by 2040. At the close of the trustees' seventy-five-year projection period in 2080, Part B transfers from general revenue will consume more than 24 percent of nonentitlement revenues.[4]

Prior to its full implementation, the Medicare Part D prescription drug benefit accounted for less than one-tenth of 1 percent of federal nonentitlement revenues. With the onset of full benefits in 2006, the share of nonentitlement tax receipts required to fund Part D rose significantly, and it will

---

4. For these calculations we treat as revenue all premium payments. We note here, however, that approximately 12 percent of Part B premium revenues represent the federal share of Part B premiums paid by the states for citizens on Medicaid. Thus, our estimated general-revenue transfers are a lower bound on the required level of such transfers.

continue to rise rapidly throughout the full seventy-five-year projection period. In 2020, less than fifteen years from now, the trustees project that Part D will require general-revenue transfers equal to 6.4 percent of nonentitlement tax receipts. By the end of the seventy-five-year projection period, more than 15 percent of nonentitlement revenues will be required to cover its projected deficits.

Taken together, Medicare Parts B and D will require general-revenue transfers of just over 11 percent in 2006. The share of the federal nonentitlement revenues required to maintain the projected level of Parts B and D benefits will rise rapidly, so that by 2020, more than 17 percent of all nonentitlement revenues must be transferred. The level of general-revenue transfers will reach 29 percent by 2040. At the close of the trustees' seventy-five-year projection period, paying for these projected benefits will require almost 40 percent of all federal nonentitlement revenues.

The required general-revenue transfers, if met with no change in taxation other than the increased payroll taxes required to balance the Medicare Part A budget, will result in non-Medicare federal expenditures as a share of the economy having to fall by roughly 40 percent. If the payroll tax rate is not increased, and general revenues are used to make up the Part A deficit in addition to the transfers required to fund Parts B and D, more than two-thirds of nonentitlement revenues will be required. Such a burden on the federal budget is the equivalent of a two-thirds reduction in non-Medicare expenditures.

A two-thirds reduction in the role of the federal government outside Medicare seems unlikely. Accordingly, as a benchmark, we will proceed by assuming that the nonentitlement role of the federal government should remain at its current share of the economy. We accomplish this by holding general-revenue transfers to Medicare as a share of GDP constant at their 2006 level. We then have an estimate of the current share of GDP that finances non-Medicare federal programs, which we then also hold constant. Using the projections of GDP from the *2006 Medicare Trustees Report*, we calculate the nonentitlement revenues that would be required to maintain non-Medicare programs. The sum of those revenues and projected general-revenue transfers to Medicare becomes our estimate of the level of nonentitlement revenues required to maintain the current share of the federal government in the economy and to cover the projected Medicare shortfalls.

FIGURE 3-3

AVERAGE TAX RATE INCREASE REQUIRED TO
MAINTAIN NONENTITLEMENT EXPENDITURES
Part A Deficits Financed with Payroll Taxes

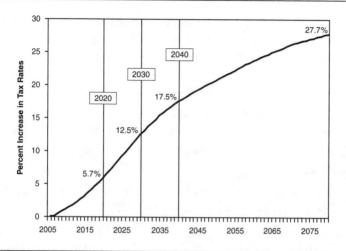

SOURCE: Authors' estimates.

The ratio of the estimated level of federal nonentitlement revenues
required to maintain the role of non-Medicare programs to the projected
level of nonentitlement revenues yields the percentage change in tax revenues required to keep the government at its current size and still able to
pay current-law projected Medicare benefits.

Taking the year 2006 as the base, and assuming that nonentitlement
revenue remains at its twenty-five-year average of 11.8 percent of GDP,
figure 3-3 shows the percentage increase in non–payroll-tax federal revenues required to pay for Medicare Parts B and D and maintain non-
Medicare federal spending.[5] The figure does not contain the entire increase
in taxation, since it assumes that Part A deficits would be covered by

---

5. To keep the analysis concentrated on Medicare and its future, we ignore the
increasing transfers that will be required if no changes are enacted in Social Security.
Thus, even if the revenues are found to fund the trustees' projected Medicare spending, Social Security transfers will still consume an ever-increasing share of the remaining nonentitlement revenues.

increases in HI payroll taxes. Nonetheless, the required tax increases are significant. In 2020, nonentitlement revenues will have to rise by almost 6 percent just to cover the projected Parts B and D shortfalls and maintain the government's non-Medicare share of GDP. By 2030, they will have to rise by more than 12 percent, by 2040 by more than 17 percent, and by the end of the seventy-five-year projection period, they must rise by almost 28 percent.

## The Pure Taxation Solution to Paying for All Projected Medicare Benefits

It is traditional in the provision of health care in the non-Medicare market to divide total expenditures into two distinct parts: in-hospital insurance and out-of-hospital insurance. We will adopt this same division in our discussion of Medicare. Moreover, this division is especially relevant for Medicare because its financing is separated in exactly this way: HI payroll taxes are meant to pay for Part A, while Parts B and D—outpatient medical insurance and prescription drugs—are by law paid for with a combination of premiums and general-revenue transfers. We have estimated the change in payroll taxes and general-revenue taxation that would allow the payment of projected benefits, assuming that current-law benefits and the setting of premiums remain intact.

From the perspective of Part A, we assumed above that all future projected deficits would be made up for with increases in the payroll tax. We constructed figure 3-1 using the trustees' projected HI cost rate expressed in terms of taxable payroll. From the perspective of Parts B and D, we allowed the remainder of federal government expenditures to maintain their share of the economy so that all the increases in Parts B and D expenditures must be paid for by increases in the government nonentitlement income.

To express the tax increases required to pay for future Medicare shortfalls in a consistent way, we do away with the assumption that the Part A deficits are separately financed through increases in HI payroll taxation. Rather, we now assume that the HI payroll tax rate remains at its current level of 2.9 percent of payroll and let all projected Medicare deficits, including the projected Part A deficit, be financed through general-revenue transfers. This approach allows us to present a more complete picture of the tax impact of the projected deficits inherent in current Medicare.

Figure 3-4 shows the percentage increase in federal nonentitlement revenues that would be required to make the necessary transfers to fund all projected Medicare deficits and allow the non-Medicare federal government to remain at its 2006 share of GDP. In less than fifteen years, in 2020, the Part A deficit's share of nonentitlement revenues, at the current payroll tax rate, will rise from essentially zero to 4.1 percent. The share consumed by Parts B and D will rise from its current level of 11.4 percent to 17.1 percent, resulting in a 2020 total transfer to Medicare of 21.2 percent of nonentitlement revenues. This increase in budget share will require a 9.6 percent increase in all federal tax rates by 2020, if other expenditures are to remain at their current share of the economy.

FIGURE 3-4

**AVERAGE TAX RATE INCREASE REQUIRED TO MAINTAIN NONENTITLEMENT EXPENDITURES**

**Part A Payroll Tax Rate Remains at Current Level**

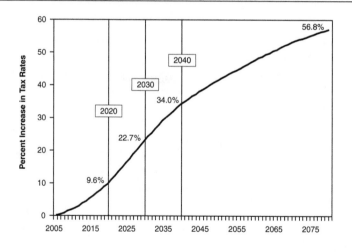

SOURCE: Authors' estimates.

Over the past twenty-five years, revenue from personal income taxation has averaged 14.38 percent of personal income. Thus, by 2020, a 9.6 percent increase will raise this average from 14.38 percent to 15.76 percent, by

2030 to 17.64 percent, and by 2040 to 19.26 percent. Finally, at the end of the seventy-five-year trustees' projection period, the average taxation of personal income will have risen from 14.38 percent of personal income to 22.55 percent.

Perhaps an easier way to understand the magnitude of the tax changes necessary to fund the projected cost of current Medicare is to express them in terms of the payroll tax rate. Figure 3-5 shows the rates that will be required if we maintain federal non-Medicare spending at its current share of GDP, including the Part A cost rate from figure 3-1. The figure clearly shows the rising share Parts B and D take of all Medicare expenditures as the widening difference between the payroll taxes that will be required, but not currently legislated, to fund Part A, the lower line in the figure, and all of Medicare, the upper line.

To fund Medicare through payroll taxation alone will require a rate of 5.57 percent in less than fifteen years (that is, by 2020), almost double the current 2.9 percent rate. Further, by 2030, the Medicare payroll tax rate will have to be 9.05 percent, more than three times the current rate, and in

FIGURE 3-5

PAYROLL TAX REQUIRED TO PAY FOR PROJECTED CURRENT MEDICARE
DEFICITS AND MAINTAIN NONENTITLEMENT EXPENDITURE SHARE OF GDP

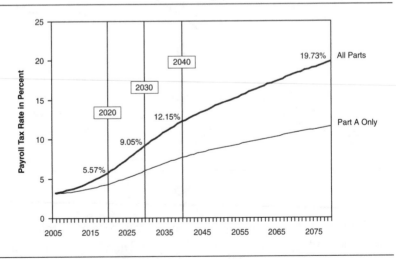

SOURCES: Authors' estimates and table VI. F2., *2006 Social Security Trustees Report.*

2040, 12.15 percent, more than four times the current rate. By the close of the seventy-five-year projection period, it will be 19.73 percent, almost seven times the current rate.

## Conclusion

It is clear from the magnitude of the Medicare funding problem that a politically feasible solution to Medicare financing will not be accomplished exclusively with taxes on the younger generation, nor expenditure cuts by Congress. If we require the young to cover the looming deficits through increased taxation, the revenue from general taxation will increase substantially from its current level of 14.4 percent of personal income to 23.1 percent. If we use payroll taxes to cover the deficits, the payroll tax will be almost 20 percent of payroll in 2080, a nearly sevenfold increase from the current 2.9 percent rate. If the Social Security deficits projected by the trustees are also covered with payroll taxation, the total payroll tax will be almost 40 percent. Taxation at the levels considered here can be expected to have incentive effects, which we have ignored. As a result, our estimates of the tax increases required are underestimates to the extent that the taxation levels have a negative effect on national output.

Thus, it seems that taxes alone will not be the choice to provide the resources required to fund a Medicare program projected to consume 11.0 percent of the country's GDP by the close of the trustees' seventy-five-year projection period. If we choose not to solve Medicare's long-run funding problem by making the young pay or by reducing the role of the federal government in the economy, what can be accomplished by transferring some or all of the cost to the elderly? In chapter 4, we address this issue.

# 4

# Paying for Projected Medicare Expenditures: Making the Elderly Pay

An alternative to using taxation of workers' income to pay for the increased cost of retirees' use of Medicare would be to impose increased premiums on the elderly to make up for some or all of the projected financing shortfalls. Such a change would alter the generational distribution of who pays, increasing the share paid by the retired generation and decreasing that of the working generation.

If we assume that increased HI payroll taxation is imposed to cover the projected Medicare Part A shortfalls, any increase in premiums would only apply to Parts B and D. However, any serious reform would put all three parts of Medicare together and apply a single premium that reflects the share of expenditures to be borne by participants.[1] In the following analysis, we leave Medicare's structure unchanged. We begin by estimating the increase in premium income that would be required to cover the projected deficits for Parts B and D, subject to the same assumptions concerning the GDP share of non-Medicare federal expenditures we used in chapter 3. Then, we estimate the Part A premium that would be required if the current level of payroll taxation were to remain unchanged and premium payments were introduced as a means of paying for projected Part A deficits.

---

1. Currently, for Parts B and D, participants' share of the cost through premium payments is only 25 percent, while their share of Part A cost is zero. A reform that made the program comprehensive has no implication, in and of itself, for the share participants would pay of its total cost.

## Using Premiums to Pay for Projected Medicare Parts B and D

In figure 4-1 we show the premiums required to cover the projected Part B
expenditures, assuming that the general-revenue transfer to Part B remains
fixed at its 2006 share of GDP.[2] As a baseline, Part B premiums now account
for 25 percent of total expenditures and are the same across beneficiaries of
all ages. The premiums are set in the fall of each year at 25 percent of
expected per-capita Part B expenditures.[3] The Medicare Modernization Act
of 2003 altered the Part B premium determination by introducing limited

FIGURE 4-1

PREMIUMS AS A SHARE OF MEDICARE PART B EXPENDITURES

Constant Transfer Share from Nonentitlement Federal Revenues

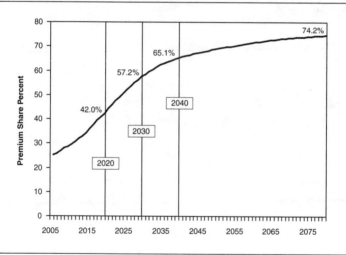

SOURCE: Authors' estimates.

2. Thus, the general-revenue transfer is allowed to grow at the same rate as GDP.
Because health-care growth exceeds GDP growth, the required transfers actually grow
faster than GDP.

3. There is the small matter of the Medicare Part B Trust Fund. The trust fund is
managed through the level of premiums and exists to allow for the payment of benefits should the forecast of expenditures be well below actual costs.

means-testing, which increases the contribution of premiums, but in a very limited sense.[4]

The share of all Part B expenditures that must be financed by premiums will rise rapidly as the expenditures rise, if the size of non-Medicare entitlement government expenditures are to remain at their 2006 level as a share of GDP in future years. By 2020, the share of all Part B expenditures paid by beneficiaries in the form of premiums will rise from its current level of 25 percent to 42 percent. Accordingly, general-revenue financing of Part B will, by 2020, have fallen to 58 percent from its current share of 75 percent. By 2030, beneficiaries will be paying for more than half, 57.2 percent, of all Part B expenditures, and by 2040, for almost two-thirds, 65.1 percent. At the close of the seventy-five-year projection period, the share will have gone up to almost three-fourths, 74.2 percent, essentially reversing the current-law-participant, general-revenue shares.

The future cost of Medicare Part D is still highly uncertain. However, requiring beneficiaries to foot the cost of any increase in Part D expenditures that exceeds the growth rate in federal nonentitlement revenue will surely result in significant increases in Part D premiums. In figure 4-2, we show the premium required when we limit the general-revenue transfer to Part D as a share of GDP to its 2006 level.

By making this transfer a fixed share of GDP, we ensure that the federal government share of GDP not devoted to Medicare entitlements remains constant. In 2006, Part D premiums were expected to account for just over 20 percent of projected total expenditures. This is expected to rise to 22.8 percent by 2015.[5] For the estimates presented in figure 4-2,

---

4. The 2003 MMA introduced a limited means-testing of premiums. However, the level of the means-testing threshold—$80,000 adjusted gross income for an individual and $160,000 adjusted gross income for a couple—has limited impact on the share of Part B expenditures covered by premiums.

5. The premium revenue for Part D comes from two sources. The first is participants who are not eligible for Medicaid. Second, for those who are eligible for Medicaid—the dual-eligibles—the states are expected to return to the federal treasury some or all of the savings they incur because of the federal subsidy to these beneficiaries. Our projections assume that these transfers actually occur. Also, because our projections fail to account for the tax burden on the citizens of the various states that may be imposed by the transfers from the states to the federal government, they are underestimates of the level of the total government—that is, federal plus state—share of health care.

FIGURE 4-2

**PREMIUMS AS A SHARE OF MEDICARE PART D EXPENDITURES**
**Constant Transfer Share from Nonentitlement Federal Revenues**

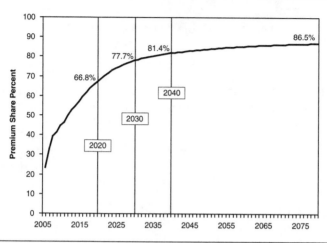

SOURCE: Authors' estimates.

we have assumed that the base premium income remains at 22.8 percent of expenditures for the entire projection period.

When Medicare beneficiaries pay for the projected shortfalls through premium increases, premiums as a share of total expenditures for Part D rise much more rapidly than as a share of total Part B expenditures. Moreover, the projected terminal value of the share of premiums to total Part D expenditures exceeds the Part B terminal value. Both of these observations result from the fact that prescription drug prices and usage have been rising faster than other health-care costs. This is evident in the rapid rise in the share of all Part D expenditures that would have to be paid with premiums if the share of federal nonentitlement income that is transferred to Part D is assumed to remain at its 2006 level. From the 2006 level of less than 21 percent, the share of Part D expenditures that would be financed by premiums rises to almost two-thirds by 2020. The share is greater than three-fourths, 77.7 percent, by 2030, and more than four-fifths, 81.4 percent, by 2040. At the close of the seventy-five-year projection period, 86.5 percent of all Part D expenditures will be paid by beneficiaries if projected Part D deficits are financed with premium increases.

What will be the total financial burden on the retired population of these projections? Figure 4-3 shows the percentage of projected Social Security benefits that our estimated premiums will consume, for workers with scaled medium and high career earnings who retire at the normal retirement age as specified by current law.[6]

FIGURE 4-3

**PREMIUMS AS A SHARE OF PROJECTED SOCIAL SECURITY BENEFITS**
Constant Transfer Share of Federal Nonentitlement Revenues to Parts B and D
Part A Payroll Tax Rates Always Equal the Part A Cost Rate

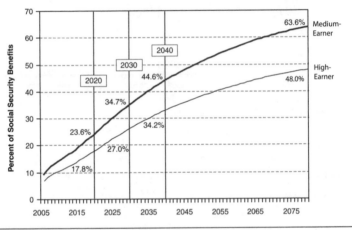

SOURCES: Authors' estimates. Transfer fixed at 2006 share of GDP from Table III.A2., *2006 Medicare Trustees Report*. New retirees' Social Security benefits from Table VI. F10., *Social Security Trustees Report*.

For a frame of reference, we use the estimate from the *2006 Medicare Trustees Report* that the Parts B and D premiums will consume 7.4 percent and 9.8 percent, respectively, of the Social Security benefits in 2006 for workers with high and medium lifetime earnings. If the projected Parts B and D deficits are covered by premiums paid by participants, these shares will rise rapidly, so that by 2020, they will be 17.8 percent and 23.6 percent, respectively, and by 2030, 27.0 percent and 34.7 percent, respec-

---

6. The Social Security benefit amounts are taken from the *2006 Social Security Trustees Report*, table VI.F10.

tively. At the end of the seventy-five-year projection period, the premiums will consume almost half of high-earner Social Security benefits and almost two-thirds of medium-earner benefits.

### Using Premiums to Pay for Projected Medicare Part A Deficits

What would be the effect of using premiums to pay for the projected Medicare Part A deficits? Figure 4-4 shows the share of projected Part A expenditures that would be paid with premiums if the current payroll tax rate were to remain at its current 2.9 percent level.

FIGURE 4-4

**PREMIUMS AS A SHARE OF MEDICARE PART A EXPENDITURES**
**Constant Transfer Share from Nonentitlement Federal Revenues**

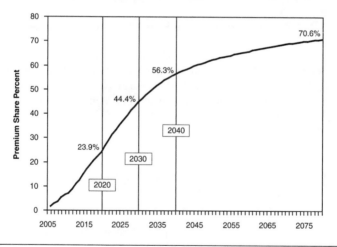

SOURCE: Authors' estimates.

The imposition of Part A premiums, combined with the premiums estimated for Parts B and D, makes elderly beneficiaries responsible for all the increased Medicare transfers in excess of the current share of the federal nonentitlement revenues being transferred. Since Part A was essentially self-supporting in 2005, premiums would be zero, but, as figure 4-4 shows, they would be positive in 2006 and would rise rapidly as the deficits grow. They would account for almost one-fourth of Part A expenditures by 2020, more than 40 percent by 2030, and well more than half by 2040. At the close of the seventy-five-year projection period, premiums would account for more than 70 percent of Part A expenditures.

## Using Premiums to Pay for All Projected Medicare Deficits

If the elderly are required to pay for all projected Medicare deficits in the form of premiums, they will end up paying for 70–86 percent of Parts A, B, and D expenditures by the end of the seventy-five-year projection period. This can be expected to place a substantial burden on elderly income. Figure 4-5 shows the projected total premium burden as a share of projected Social Security benefits for scaled medium and high career earners who retire at the normal retirement age, as specified by current law.

FIGURE 4-5

PARTS A, B, AND D PREMIUMS AS A SHARE OF PROJECTED SOCIAL SECURITY BENEFITS
Medicare Transfer Is a Constant Share of Federal Nonentitlement Revenues
Part A Payroll Taxes Remain at Current Level

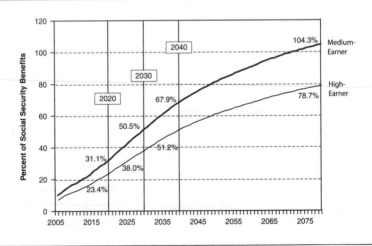

SOURCES: Authors' estimates. Transfer fixed at 2006 share of GDP from Table III.A2., *2006 Medicare Trustees Report.* New retirees' Social Security benefits from Table VI. F10., *Social Security Trustees Report.*

If premium increases are used to cover the projected revenue shortfalls for all parts of Medicare, the share of retirees' Social Security benefit checks going to premium revenues will rise rapidly. By 2020, premiums will consume 23.4 percent of a high-earner's and 31.1 percent of a medium-earner's benefit. This burden will continue to rise, and, at the close of the seventy-five-year projection period, Medicare premiums will consume more than three-fourths of the Social Security benefits for high-earning individuals and more than 100 percent for retirees who had medium lifetime earnings.

## Conclusion

The levels of premiums required to fund the future funding shortfalls of current Medicare make it clear that the program's financing problems cannot be solved exclusively with premiums paid by the elderly. A reformed Medicare that fixes the level of general-revenue transfers at their current share of GDP and requires users to pick up the difference implies premiums that would ultimately cover more than 70 percent of total expenditures. Such premium levels would consume most of a Social Security recipient's benefit check, more than three-fourths of a high-earner's check, and more than 100 percent of a medium-earner's check. Even though many of the elderly are wealthier than the younger generation, their earnings plus Social Security benefits are considerably less than the income of the working population. Thus, the financial burden of the premiums we forecast would be excessive.

From chapter 3, we know that requiring the young to cover the looming deficits through increased taxation implies that the revenue from taxation of workers will have to rise dramatically—an increase from the current level of 14.4 percent of personal income to 23.1 percent—or require payroll taxation of almost 20 percent. Thus, neither taxes nor premiums alone can provide the resources required to fund a Medicare program that is projected to consume 11 percent of the country's GDP by the close of the trustees' seventy-five-year projection period.

The scale of the Medicare problem has elicited a number of suggested reforms. In the following four chapters we analyze five of them, projecting their respective impacts on the level of Medicare expenditures and on the program's ultimate financial status. These impacts are of critical importance to the long-run sustainability of Medicare, not just on the level of Medicare expenditures, but in terms of the overall rate of growth of health-care expenditures. In reviewing them, it is important to keep in mind that reforms that affect the current level of expenditures but not the growth of the health-care sector will not solve the Medicare funding problem in the very long run. Ultimately, the growth of health care as a share of the economy is the choice of the population. As incomes rise, individuals may desire to increase the share of that income they spend on health care.

These choices only concern us because, given the current structure of Medicare, the elderly population it serves does not care what health care costs. We can rest assured that if the buyers of a product do not care what they pay for it, the suppliers of the product can be expected to take full advantage of that fact. Further, a system where the direct consumers are not concerned about price requires extensive and expensive oversight, a fact of life for those in the health-care industry as they cope with the extensive paperwork required for reimbursement. On the other hand, if a reform could be found that resulted in consumers caring about price, they would perform the oversight themselves, and outside monitoring would be unnecessary.

# 5

# Scoring Medicare Reform I:
# The Medicare Commission

The imposition of tax increases on working generations or of premium payments on the elderly by themselves to solve Medicare's financing shortfalls are measures that seem unlikely ever to be enacted. What, then, can or should be done to remedy the problem? There are two principal issues that any reform must resolve. First, we must determine if the problem is that we are consuming too much health care throughout our lives. If so, reforms should be evaluated on the basis of their effectiveness in reducing overconsumption and how any such measures would affect the long-run sustainability of the reformed Medicare. Second, we must ask, regardless of the level of health care desired by the population, how should the costs of it be distributed across generations?

In chapter 3, we applied the trustees' projections of Medicare's finances to derive the funding levels they implied. Our analysis ignored the question of how those levels of funding would affect the preretirement saving and labor-supply decisions of citizens. We simply assumed the level of GDP projected by the trustees would remain the same no matter how the projected Medicare deficits were financed.

Implicitly, we assumed that individual behavior would be unaffected by the level of taxation we forecast would be required to finance Medicare deficits—the same assumption implicit in producing both the Social Security and Medicare trustees reports. We further assumed that individual behavior would be unaffected if, rather than taxation, premiums were imposed on the retired generation to pay for the future deficits. The imposition of such premiums would take for granted that workers had prepared themselves financially to pay them after retirement.

In this and the next three chapters, we evaluate proposals that have been suggested by ourselves and others to deal with the rising costs of health care and their effects on Medicare financing. In each case, we estimate the impact of the enactment of the proposed changes on the long-run sustainability of the program from a financial point of view.

There are two levels of Medicare reform. The first set of reforms—the majority of them—deals with who pays for health care and essentially does not address, at least not directly, the projected levels of consumption. These reforms are the subject of chapters 5 and 6. The second, smaller class of reforms involves means-testing and the elimination of "first-dollar coverage" and deals with altering the projections of future Medicare spending. These are evaluated in chapters 7 and 8.

### General Issues in Medicare Reform

Average Medicare spending, along with average health-care spending among individuals of less than retirement age, has grown faster than per-capita GDP for the last fifty years. The relative growth in health-care spending has been attributed to the payment mechanisms in place, technological change, rising income, and an assortment of other factors. In chapters 3 and 4 we identified the changes in tax collections and premium payments that will be necessary to pay for Medicare as projected by the trustees. For those exercises, however, we took the trustees' projections of Medicare costs as given. We did not address how Medicare, and, for that matter, how health-care delivery in general might change in the future.

Based on the 2006 trustees report, Medicare spending is projected to account for 8.5 percent of GDP by mid-century and 10.99 percent by 2080. But Medicare is only part of the health-care pie. The same procedures that produced the estimates for Medicare indicate that medical care for all Americans will account for 35.7 percent of GDP by 2050 and 42.8 percent by 2080. As we mentioned in the previous chapter, if these estimates do not seem plausible, then maybe they are not.

However, we must step back and ask, what does not seem plausible? Is it implausible that health-care spending will be more than 35 percent of GDP in 2050, or that the government will continue to pay for at least half of that spending? There have been plenty of pronouncements in the past that certain predicted outcomes would not or could not happen, with those outcomes having been realized after all. When we think about Medicare reform, are we trying to devise a payment system that somehow stems the growth in health-care spending as a share of GDP, or are we reallocating who pays or how we pay for the same expected expenditures? Trying to reduce the amount of health care each Medicare beneficiary consumes during his or her retirement, as compared to spending as it is currently projected, will require a comprehensive reform that also addresses individual spending prior to retirement. Most reform proposals reallocate who pays for retirement medical care and when that payment occurs.

Before we present our evaluation of Medicare reform proposals, we should go over our ground rules for scoring them. We begin by taking the *2006 Medicare Trustees Report* projections for expenditures and revenues as given. In projecting the general-revenue requirements of Medicare Parts B and D, the trustees treat the premium revenues as net income to the system. For our scoring of the Medicare reform proposals, we adopt this same approach. In reality, however, the elderly and handicapped who are on Medicaid get some or all of their Part B and D premiums paid for by the government, either state or federal. Thus, the estimated general-revenue transfers required both for Medicare as it is now and the various reforms to Medicare we are about to consider are understated. For our purposes, premium income is assumed to remain at the current percentages of Parts B and D spending across all reforms. Finally, in order to distinguish Medicare as it currently is structured from the several reforms we consider, we will always refer to it as "Current Medicare."

## The Medicare Commission Reform

We begin our discussion of Medicare reform with perhaps the most politically feasible option, suggested by the National Bipartisan Commission on the Future of Medicare (1999).[1] While the commission predated the

---

1. Senator John Breaux and Representative Bill Thomas were the commission's statutory and administrative chairmen, respectively.

establishment of Medicare Part D, the incorporation of a prescription plan was part of its plan. The commission recommended that all Medicare be combined into a single system with a premium covering all aspects of health care. The principal elements of this plan are described below.

1. Private health providers would compete with a government-run, fee-for-service plan. Individuals would choose between a private plan or the government plan, with the private plan's premiums paid by a combination of individual and government funds.

2. A standard benefits package equivalent to Current Medicare would be offered.

3. Beneficiaries would pay a premium equaling 12 percent of per-capita costs. If they chose a package with a price less than 85 percent of the national weighted average cost, they would pay no premium. If they chose one above the national weighted average cost, they would pay the entire difference in cost.[2]

4. The basic fee-for-service plan would have a deductible of $400, to be indexed to per-capita Medicare cost. In 1999, the year the commission's report was released, per-capita cost of the sum of Medicare Parts A and B was $5,502. The 2006 Medicare Trustees Report projected these costs as $10,685 for 2006, so the deductible in 2006 dollars would have been $777.[3]

5. A coinsurance payment of 10 percent would be charged for home health services, laboratory services, and certain other services not currently subject to coinsurance, but no coinsurance would be charged for hospital stays and preventive care.[4]

_____

2. For purposes of calculating the national weighted average cost, only the cost of standard benefits is counted.

3. The sum of Parts A, B, and D deductibles for Current Medicare is $1,326 ($952 for Part A, $124 for Part B, and $250 for Part D).

4. The coinsurance for Current Medicare is 20 percent for Part B and 25 percent for Part D up to the initial benefit limit; then 100 percent to the next limit; then 5 percent. For current Part A, coinsurance is defined in terms of the deductible rather than actual charges. Part A coinsurance kicks in after day sixty of an illness and is

6. The age of Medicare eligibility would be raised to coincide with the normal retirement age as defined by Social Security legislation, currently sixty-six years of age and scheduled to increase by two months a year beginning in 2017, until reaching sixty-seven years of age in 2022.

7. In any year in which the general-fund contributions to Medicare are projected to exceed 40 percent of annual Medicare outlays, the trustees would be required to notify Congress that the program was in danger of becoming programmatically insolvent.[5]

A few years after the commission's report was released, Congress passed the 2003 Medicare Modernization Act (MMA) that created the current-law prescription drug benefit. Other aspects of the MMA enhanced the competition between HMOs and traditional fee-for-service Medicare through changes in Part C, now called Medicare Advantage. Medicare Advantage C is an array of health-care delivery options available to Medicare beneficiaries in addition to traditional fee-for-service, including health maintenance organizations and preferred provider organizations. In 2006, approximately 13 percent of Medicare beneficiaries were enrolled under Medicare Advantage.

Some, or perhaps even much, of the reform suggested by the commission has thus been implemented, with the exception of increasing the age of eligibility from the current level of sixty-five to sixty-seven years. To evaluate the effect of the commission's proposal on Medicare's projected funding shortfalls, we must analyze its effect on the trustees' projections.

---

25 percent of the deductible (which was $952 in 2006) for each of the next thirty days, and then 50 percent of the deductible per day thereafter.

5. The 2003 Medicare Modernization Act set the trigger for informing the president of potential program insolvency at 45 percent. Specifically, if projected Medicare expenditures are expected to require general-revenue transfers of more than 45 percent of total expenditures within a seven-year horizon for two consecutive years, the trustees are required to send an alert to the president, and the president is required to produce proposals to Congress to rectify the problem. See chapter 2 for further discussion.

As noted above, the commission's proposal combined all parts of Medicare into a single unit and applied a single premium initially set at 12 percent of per-capita expenditures. As an initial estimate of the proposal's effect on Medicare shortfalls, we look at the projections from the *2006 Medicare Trustees Report*. To make the current projections relevant we combine all parts of Medicare into a single unit. Given that "Commission Medicare" will include all eligible individuals ages sixty-six and over, the appropriate enrollment figure is Part A enrollment as projected by the trustees, less the effect of an increase in the age of eligibility to the current Social Security normal retirement age of sixty-six and the gradual increase in the age of eligibility that will begin in 2015.[6]

So that no current beneficiaries lose coverage, we estimate the cost of Commission Medicare by restricting new entrants to the program beginning in 2006 based on the Social Security normal retirement age and its progression.[7] We assume that the percentage reduction in Part B expenditures attributable to the sixty-five-year-old Medicare population will be the same for Part D, since there is no history for Part D. We then adjust these smaller expenditures to account for the fact that Commission Medicare is a single package in which all those eligible are enrolled.

The commission envisioned that the adoption of its proposal would reduce the *long-term* rate of growth of Medicare by one percentage point per year. However, there is good reason to believe this is overly optimistic. First, the commission deductible is less than half that of Current Medicare. Second, the commission coinsurance is smaller than that of Current Medicare. Third, the MMA results in a Medicare that has many of the components of the commission reform. Fourth, while it may seem that increasing the age of eligibility would have a significant effect on cost, sixty-five- and sixty-six-year-olds currently make up less than 2 percent of Medicare expenditures. While this share will rise with the retirement of the baby boomers, it is never expected to exceed 5 percent of Part A and 7 percent of Part B at any time in the

---

6. For 2006, the trustees estimated that Part A enrollment would exceed Part B enrollment by 6.1 percent and Part D enrollment by 43 percent, although this latter projection had already been exceeded by the time their report was released.

7. Estimates of the Medicare expenditures of sixty-five- and sixty-six-year-olds are derived from the Continuous Medicare History Sample file (CMHS; U.S. Department of Health and Human Services 2004).

trustees' seventy-five-year projection period. Thus, we believe that the projections from the *2006 Medicare Trustees Report*, adjusted for the age of eligibility, form the basis for an estimate of the cost of Commission Medicare.

Figure 5-1 shows the transfers required to fund Commission Medicare and Current Medicare as shares of federal nonentitlement revenues. While Commission Medicare improves the long-run outlook, it does not come close to solving Medicare's solvency problem. The improvement in finances is due entirely to the increased age of eligibility. The commission's proposal of a premium equal to 12 percent of total Medicare is not a factor, since the current premiums on Parts B and D are already 13 percent of total Medicare expenditures, including Part A. Commission Medicare, with its increased age of eligibility, still leaves us with having to transfer more than 20 percent of nonentitlement revenues to Medicare in less than fifteen years, more than 31 percent by 2030, and more than 43 percent by 2040. At the close of the seventy-five-year projection period, Commission Medicare would require that we transfer more than 65 percent of all nonentitlement revenues to Medicare.

FIGURE 5-1

**COMMISSION MEDICARE REQUIRED TRANSFERS**
**Percent Nonentitlement Federal Taxes**

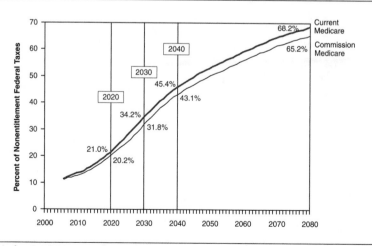

SOURCE: Authors' estimates.

NOTE: Federal nonentitlement taxes are estimated to be 11.8 percent of GDP, the twenty-five-year average.

The magnitude of the required general-revenue transfers has not escaped the attention of Congress, as mentioned previously in connection with the MMA's 45 percent general-revenue funding trigger. Figure 5-2 shows the general-revenue share projections for both Current Medicare and Commission Medicare.[8]

According to the figure, Commission Medicare results in a very small improvement to the share of expenditures that must be financed with general revenues. The initial effect is zero, because we assumed that the increased age of eligibility would not apply to those who reached sixty-five years of age before the reform was begun. The later improvement is a result of the elimination of two years of beneficiaries. Clearly, the solution to creating a Medicare that will be financially sound cannot be found in the commission's recommendations.

FIGURE 5-2

GENERAL-REVENUE SHARE: COMMISSION VERSUS
CURRENT MEDICARE EXPENDITURES

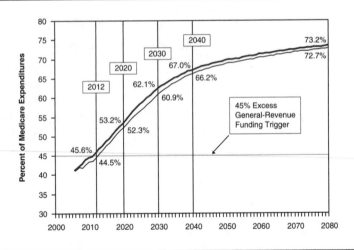

SOURCES: Authors' estimates and from Table III.A2. and Figure III.A1., *2006 Medicare Trustees Report* and Table VI.F4., *2006 Social Security Trustees Report.*

---

8. Recall that the commission recommendation was for an excess general-revenue trigger set at 40 percent of Medicare expenditures.

## Conclusion

Given the plethora of suggestions for reforming Medicare, the dearth of estimates of the contribution that any one of these reforms, if enacted, would
make toward solving the looming financial crisis is surprising. In this chapter
we have estimated the financial impact of one of these reforms. One way to
compare any suggested reform is to review its impact on the level of the transfer required at the close of the trustees' seventy-five-year projection period.
This comparison is useful because, given the assumption by the trustees that
at the close of this period health-care spending growth will be equal to the
growth rate of per-capita GDP, the shares of general revenue required to fund
Medicare will remain at the share estimated in the terminal year of the projection period.

   In figure 5-3, we show the terminal-year share of federal nonentitlement revenues required to pay for the government's share of Medicare for
Commission and Current Medicare. Commission Medicare does reduce the
level of transfers required, but by less than 5 percent. Considering that
Current Medicare will require a transfer of more than 68 percent of all

FIGURE 5-3

**TERMINAL-YEAR SHARE OF NONENTITLEMENT REVENUES:
COMMISSION VERSUS CURRENT MEDICARE**

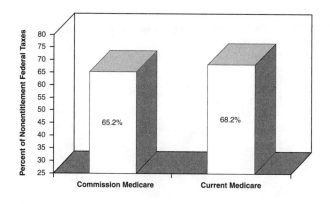

SOURCE: Authors' estimates.

federal nonentitlement revenues in 2080, the reduction in this transfer arising from Commission Medicare to just over 65 percent has little effect on the long-run sustainability of the program.

While looking at the terminal values of the required transfers reflects the long-run aspects of Commission Medicare, these values are not necessarily representative of the full benefit over the seventy-five-year projection period. The trustees summarize the impact of Medicare for the current generation in terms of the seventy-five-year unfunded liability. In Figure 5-4, we show this unfunded liability for Commission and Current Medicare. Current Medicare has a $32.4 trillion dollar liability. Commission Medicare, which brings the age of eligibility for Medicare in line with the full retirement age of Social Security, has a liability of $30.7 trillion, paying off just under $1.7 trillion of Current Medicare's liability.

While figure 5-4 is similar to figure 5-3, where we show required general-revenue transfers for Commission Medicare and Current Medicare the magnitudes of the relative reductions in unfunded liability are almost identical to the relative reductions in terminal-year transfers in figure 5-3.

FIGURE 5-4
SEVENTY-FIVE-YEAR UNFUNDED LIABILITY:
COMMISSION VERSUS CURRENT MEDICARE

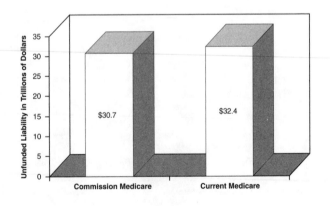

SOURCES: Authors' estimates and table V.E2., *2006 Medicare Trustees Report.*

Commission Medicare's terminal-year-transfer share of federal nonentitlement revenues is 95.6 percent that of Current Medicare, while Commission Medicare's seventy-five-year unfunded liability is 94.8 percent that of Current Medicare.

# 6

# Scoring Medicare Reform II: Fixing Technology at Retirement

Contrasting retirees' Medicare benefits to their Social Security benefits provides a convenient way of introducing Medicare reforms that constrain the growth rate in per-capita transfers. Once initial Social Security benefit amounts are determined for retirees, future benefits grow through retirement with a cost-of-living adjustment. Medicare is different in that the value of the insurance it provides grows throughout a retiree's life with advances in medical technology and with the rising cost of care associated with older ages. In this chapter, we consider two ways of making Medicare more like Social Security in terms of the growth in benefits after sixty-five years of age.

For the computation of a retiree's Social Security benefits, past taxable earnings are inflated by a wage index so that all past earnings are placed on a current real-wage basis. However, once these benefits are determined at retirement, future benefits are fixed in purchasing power through price-indexing. Each new group of retirees receives larger benefits than the previous cohort due to wage growth between cohorts, although, once again, when a cohort reaches retirement age, its benefits are fixed in real terms. In a similar way, beginning Medicare benefits for new retirees increase with the expansion of health-care usage—that is, they are escalated by health-care cost growth, just as initial Social Security benefits are escalated by wage growth. There, however, the similarity ends. Medicare benefits continue to increase with health-care cost growth throughout beneficiaries' lifetimes regardless of the year in which they retire, whereas increases in real wages in the economy have no effect on retirees' Social Security benefits once they are awarded.

Figure 6-1 illustrates the dramatic difference between Medicare's and Social Security's respective cost-paths. In this figure, projected Social Security and Medicare costs are indexed to their respective shares of GDP as of 2006. By 2080, Social Security's costs as a share of GDP will be about 50 percent higher than its share in 2006. Medicare's projected share of GDP will be 242 percent higher. Given that Medicare and Social Security share the same demographics, almost all of the difference between the two projections comprises growth in health-care spending in excess of real price-level changes. As we have already seen, the current financing arrangement will result in much of this increased consumption by Medicare beneficiaries being paid for by taxpayers.

FIGURE 6-1

**SOCIAL SECURITY AND MEDICARE: PERCENTAGE OF GDP INDEXED TO 2006**

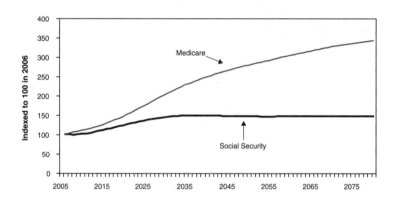

SOURCE: Authors' estimates.

One possible reform, then, would be to adjust Medicare's benefits after retirement using a method more like the price-indexing of postretirement Social Security. With such a reform, initial Medicare benefits would rise with the expansion of health-care usage, as they do now. Once Medicare eligibility age is reached, however, future benefit levels would allow for the anticipated age-related rise in spending, but would be fixed in real terms.

This reform would be implemented by fixing the basic coverage at the time of retirement to follow the age-benefit profile that exists in that year. As standards for health coverage expand, new retirees would get this new coverage in their initially awarded age-benefit profile, while existing retirees would be required to pay for it. Given that our aggregate Medicare estimates are derived from the *2006 Medicare Trustees Report*, the progression of spending by birth cohort is smooth, though technological advances, and their costs, may be discrete in nature. In our stylized estimates, each new cohort of retirees receives the technology that exists when they retire and pays for any technological innovations introduced during their retirement through increased premiums or cost-sharing.

A still more drastic reform would be fixing the benefit structure as of a given year, say 2011, the year the first baby boomers reach sixty-five years of age, but only allowing subsequent retirees an initial benefit increase that equals real per-capita GDP growth applied to the 2011 technology, rather than real per-capita health-care expenditure growth. Further, subsequent growth during retirement would be restricted to general price-level growth applied to the age-spending profile. This reform would result in the growth in real cost of Medicare to taxpayers as a share of GDP being much closer to the growth in Social Security. If the trustees' projected path for Current Medicare expenditures is unaffected by the reduced subsidy to the elderly, then future retirees would be responsible for a greater share of their retirement health-care consumption. As a result, they would need to save more while in the labor force than they would if the current arrangement persists.[1]

Compared to Current Medicare, both of these proposals are benefit reductions, in that they require retirees to pay for all growth in the age-spending distribution in excess of price-level effects. Thus, retirees pay a growing share of their health-care expenses as they age. Assuming that who pays does not affect expenditures, these reforms change the distribution of who pays from workers to retirees. Based on the alternative ways of constraining Medicare growth that we have touched on above, we now provide

---

1. This reform is similar to one suggested by Laurence J. Kotlikoff and Scott Burns (2003) whereby after the base year, benefits grow at the level of real wage growth.

some accounting for the effects of each alternative on the program's cost. These are best illustrated by considering how they change the age-spending profiles for several successive groups of new retirees as compared to Current Medicare.

In contrast to Social Security, Current Medicare benefits are unrelated to past earnings; the benefit package is identical for all retirees, regardless of the year of retirement; and, importantly, benefits grow both with relatively faster growth in health-care prices and with rising quantity of care. Given Current Medicare's projected growth, the value of its lifetime insurance coverage grows relative to past earnings for all birth cohorts of retirees, whereas Social Security benefits as a share of past earnings are relatively constant across all future cohorts of retirees. That is, each new group of entrants into the Medicare program will receive benefits over their lifetimes that are a larger share of their lifetime earnings and compensation than the groups of retirees who came before them. Current Medicare's "replacement" rate is, therefore, rising for each new group of retirees.

Medicare reforms that fix the age-benefit profile at retirement will produce rising benefits for successive groups of retirees, but not at the same rate as the current program, which, as noted, allows benefits to grow during retirement with changes in health-care consumption. The rate of cohort-to-cohort growth in lifetime benefits would be more like the growth in lifetime Social Security benefits across birth cohorts.

To estimate how these two ways of setting the age-benefit profile at retirement affect total spending, we first decompose total projected Medicare spending in each year by age and population. The lifetime spending pattern for an average member of a birth cohort generally rises as the retiree ages because of increasing health-care utilization at higher ages, new technology, rising prices through time, and the general rise in health-care spending, regardless of age, through time. For both of the above reforms that fix the level of benefits at retirement, implementation is the same and involves the comparison between the age-expenditure forecast based on Current Medicare and that projected under either fixed-benefit rule.

We begin with the historical average annual age-spending profiles for men and women that allow us to estimate future spending profiles for each year.[2] Figure 6-2 depicts how average spending rises with age, in the cross-section and for a particular birth cohort. We present two spending profiles adjusted to 2006 dollars: first, average annual spending by age for all Medicare beneficiaries in 2003, the solid line in the figure; and second, average annual spending at each age for members of the 1909 birth cohort as they aged from 1974, when they reached sixty-five, to 2003, when the survivors were ninety-four, the dashed line in the figure.[3] For the 2003 cross-section profile, average spending generally rises with age until individuals reach their mid-nineties and then falls. Given that this profile is based on a single year of data—a snapshot of a point in time—the concave shape is determined by the spending at each age and not by changes in health-care costs or changing technology.

The time-series profile represents the spending of the 1909 cohort, which turned sixty-five in the first year for which we have data, 1974. The surviving members of this cohort were ninety-four years of age in the last year of our data, 2003. As this series indicates, average spending of a particular cohort rises rapidly. In contrast to the cross-sectional age-spending profile for 2003, the time-series profile tracks average real spending by members of a single cohort, and thus its shape is affected by changes in the intensity of use, health-care price growth, and changing technology.

Now we can turn to the projected age-spending series.[4] The projected age-spending profiles are used to allocate aggregate spending by aged beneficiaries derived from the *2006 Medicare Trustees Report*. This way of allocating total spending to single years of age ensures that the component parts when summed together in each year are consistent with the aggregate-spending forecast.

---

2. The data used to make the forecasts are a 5 percent sample of Medicare beneficiaries in each year from 1974 to 2003 from the Continuous Medicare History Sample (CMHS); (U.S. Department of Health and Human Services 2004). The sample is constructed in such a way that we can also track Medicare reimbursements from the year an individual becomes eligible until he or she dies, or until the last year in the dataset; but for the present exercise we use the data to calculate average spending in each year by age and sex. These averaged data are used to forecast future spending profiles.

3. Prices are adjusted using the Consumer Price Index for wage earners (CPI-W) because it is the index used to calculate the cost-of-living adjustments (COLAs) for Social Security benefits.

FIGURE 6-2
BENEFICIARIES BORN IN 1909 AND THE 2003 CROSS-SECTION

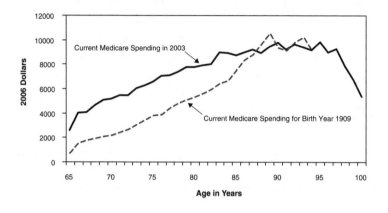

SOURCE: Authors' estimates from the Continuous Medicare History Sample.

We distinguish between the two ways of fixing the age-benefit profile at retirement by referring to the first method as Retirement Technology Medicare and the second as 2011 Technology Medicare. Retirement Technology Medicare is identified for each birth cohort as the cross-sectional age-spending profile, derived from the trustees report estimates, that exists in the year in which the cohort reaches sixty-five years of age. For all subsequent years after retirement, the profile is indexed by price-level growth. We define 2011 Technology Medicare for each birth cohort retiring in 2011 and

---

4. The predicted spending patterns are based on regressions that allow the shape of the age-spending profile to change through time. Separate weighted regressions for men and women are estimated using the average spending by age profiles for each of the years from 1974 to 2003. The dependent variable is average spending, and the independent variables are controls for each age, a time trend, and the time trend interacted with each age. The estimated coefficients are then used to predict spending for men and women at each age until 2080. Shares of spending by age in each year are derived by combining the predicted spending profiles with population counts of aged Medicare beneficiaries. These shares are then used to allocate predicted Medicare spending by aged beneficiaries using aggregate spending estimates derived from the *2006 Medicare Trustees Report*.

later as the 2011 age-spending profile, indexed by real GDP growth to the year in which the cohort reaches sixty-five years of age. This profile is likewise indexed by price-level growth for all years after retirement.

Figure 6-3 depicts the projected spending profiles for the oldest members of the baby boom generation—those born in 1946 who will reach age sixty-five in 2011. For this birth cohort, Retirement Technology Medicare and 2011 Technology Medicare are the same. As a point of reference, the Current Medicare series tracks the projected real 2006 value of their spending as they age based on our allocation of total spending on aged beneficiaries as derived from the trustees report. For this birth cohort, our estimates for Current Medicare have real average annual spending peaking at almost $34,000 (in 2006 dollars) in 2041, when members of the 1946 cohort reach ninety-five years of age.

FIGURE 6-3

**SPENDING PROFILES FOR BENEFICIARIES BORN IN 1946**

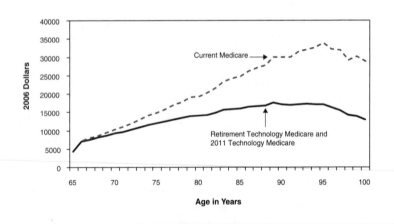

SOURCE: Authors' estimates from the Continuous Medicare History Sample.

In controlling postretirement Medicare cost growth with Retirement Technology Medicare, a retiree's benefits are essentially indexed by healthcare costs up to the age of Medicare eligibility and then required to follow the cross-sectional path indexed to price-level changes after the age of sixty-five rather than the time-series path of expenditures, defined by the age-spending profile in the year of retirement. Thus, if the cohort's Medicare transfers are limited to the technology that existed in the year its members retired, the transfers would follow the age-spending path depicted by the projected 2011 profile. As mentioned, for the birth year depicted in figure 6-3, Retirement Technology Medicare and 2011 Technology Medicare are the same. Applying either option requires that the difference between the two profiles be made up by premiums or by higher cost-sharing. Either option might affect spending incentives and, thus, total spending at each age, as well as the growth rate in spending. As a result, our estimates of the benefits of either Retirement Technology Medicare or 2011 Technology Medicare as the difference between its spending profile and the Current Medicare profile represent the maximum additional funding required from this group of retirees or, put differently, the minimum reduction in the budget transfers required to fund either Retirement Technology Medicare or 2011 Technology Medicare.[5]

Once we get beyond the 1946 cohort, Retirement Technology Medicare and 2011 Technology Medicare begin to differ, and the further we move from 2011, the greater the difference. Figure 6-4 (on the following page) shows the spending profiles facing the 1960 birth cohort under the two reforms, Retirement Technology Medicare and 2011 Technology Medicare, and under Current Medicare, again used as a point of reference. For this particular cohort, the 2011 Technology Medicare and the Retirement Technology Medicare profiles differ as the result of the fourteen years of higher growth in per-capita health-care spending than in per-capita GDP. As expected, the profile for Current Medicare has a shape similar to that for the individuals born in 1946, but because of general inflation in the cost of health care, the highest annual spending is almost $46,000 at ninety-five years of age in 2055, versus the $34,000 age-ninety-five spending for the 1946 cohort.

---

5. The growing difference between the Current Medicare profile and the Retirement Technology profile does not necessarily imply rising real premiums as the cohort ages. A constant annual premium amount, which takes into account the relative profiles and the life expectancy of the cohort, can be calculated. The calculation of the constant premium payments for successive birth cohorts is discussed in the next chapter.

The other two profiles in the figure reflect the transfers to which this cohort would be entitled under Retirement Technology Medicare and 2011 Technology Medicare, respectively. Recall that 2011 Technology Medicare does not completely fix the age-spending profile at its 2011 level for all future cohorts, but adjusts it by real per-capita GDP growth. This adjustment is considerably less than the one made in Retirement Technology Medicare, which lets the initial age-spending be the profile at age of retirement, implying that the initial profile is indexed by growth in health-care costs. The difference between the two profiles shows the progression of spending at each age in excess of real per-capita GDP growth for the years between 2011 and 2025, when the 1960 cohort reaches sixty-five years of age. The maximum spending for the 1960 cohort, based on the 2025 cross-sectional profile, is almost $24,000 at the age of eighty-nine.

FIGURE 6-4

**SPENDING PROFILES FOR BENEFICIARIES BORN IN 1960**

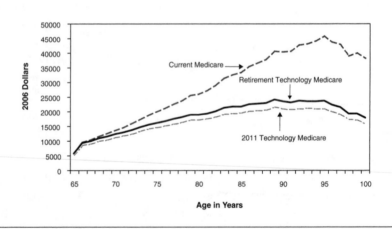

SOURCE: Authors' estimates from the Continuous Medicare History Sample.

In figure 6-5 we depict the age-spending profiles for the cohort born in 1980. This cohort turns one hundred in 2080, the last year of the trustees' seventy-five-year projection period. The relative shapes of the three profiles are again similar to those in figure 6-4, but the distance between the profiles representing Retirement Technology Medicare and 2011 Technology Medicare widens as a result of the passage of twenty more years in which real per-capita health-care spending outpaced real per-capita GDP growth. Average real spending for this cohort in 2075, when its members reach ninety-five, is almost $63,000.

FIGURE 6-5

**SPENDING PROFILES FOR BENEFICIARIES BORN IN 1980**

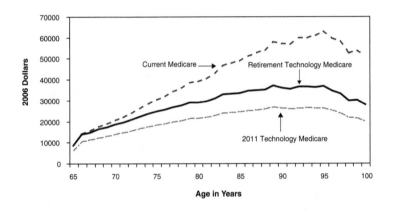

SOURCE: Authors' estimates from the Continuous Medicare History Sample.

Figure 6-6 shows the transfers required to fund Retirement Technology Medicare and Current Medicare as a share of federal nonentitlement revenues. While Retirement Technology Medicare improves the long-run outlook, Medicare's financing requirements remain sizable in the long run. The improvement is due to limiting the growth in expenditures once a cohort retires. After estimating the effects of the reform, we find a transfer of 17.1 percent of nonentitlement revenues to Medicare is necessary in less than fifteen years. It rises to more than 25 percent by 2030, and to more than one-third by 2040. At the close of the seventy-five-year projection period, Retirement Technology Medicare would require a transfer of more than 55 percent of all federal nonentitlement revenues to

FIGURE 6-6
REQUIRED TRANSFERS: RETIREMENT TECHNOLOGY
VERSUS CURRENT MEDICARE
Percent Federal Nonentitlement Revenues

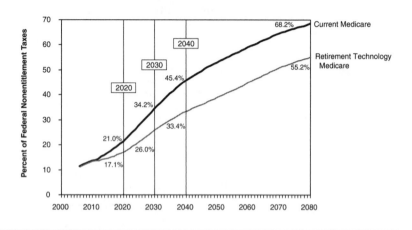

SOURCE: Authors' estimates.
NOTE: Federal nonentitlement taxes are estimated to be 11.8 percent of GDP, the twenty-five-year average.

Medicare, down from Current Medicare's 68.2 percent, but still a burden that would be difficult to bear.

Figure 6-7 shows the general-revenue share of Medicare expenditures for Retirement Technology Medicare and Current Medicare. Since we begin the reform in 2011, the year the leading edge of the baby boom becomes eligible for Medicare, the 2012 general-revenue share is almost identical for both. By 2020, however, the general-revenue share of Retirement Technology Medicare is just over 9 percent smaller than that of Current Medicare. At the close of the seventy-five-year projection period, the general-revenue share of all Medicare expenditures is only 2.5 percentage points different.

Figure 6-8 depicts the transfers required to fund 2011 Technology Medicare and Current Medicare as a share of federal nonentitlement revenues. While 2011 Technology Medicare, too, only goes part of the way in solving Medicare's long-run financing requirements, it improves the long-run outlook more than Retirement Technology Medicare does. The

FIGURE 6-7

**GENERAL-REVENUE SHARE: RETIREMENT TECHNOLOGY
VERSUS CURRENT MEDICARE EXPENDITURES**

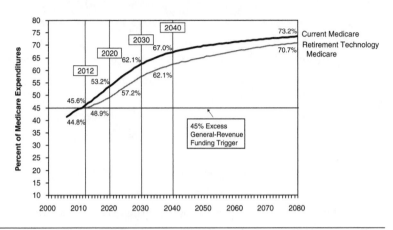

SOURCES: Authors' estimates and from Table III.A2. and Figure III.A1., *2006 Medicare Trustees Report* and Table VI.F4., *2006 Social Security Trustees Report.*

FIGURE 6-8

**REQUIRED TRANSFERS: 2011 TECHNOLOGY VERSUS CURRENT MEDICARE**
Percent Federal Nonentitlement Revenues

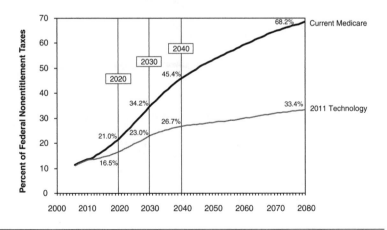

SOURCE: Authors' estimates.
NOTE: Federal nonentitlement taxes are estimated to be 11.8 percent of GDP, the twenty-five-year average.

improvement is due to limiting the growth in initial expenditures to the level of per-capita GDP growth after 2011, rather than the larger growth rate of per-capita health-care expenditures. In less than fifteen years, even this quite aggressive reform requires the transfer of 16.5 percent of nonentitlement revenues, of 23 percent by 2030, and of more than 25 percent in 2040. Importantly, at the close of the seventy-five-year projection period, 2011 Technology Medicare would require that we transfer more than one-third of all nonentitlement revenues to Medicare. While this quite drastic reform reduces the end-of-period transfer to less than half of that required for Current Medicare, the transfer of a third of all federal nonentitlement revenues may not be a sustainable solution to the program's funding problems.

Figure 6-9 shows the general-revenue share of Medicare expenditures for 2011 Technology Medicare, which indexes 2011 technology by per-capita GDP growth to the year a cohort retires and adjusts for price-level changes thereafter. As with Retirement Technology Medicare, beginning the reform in 2011 results in little difference in the 2012 general-revenue share

### FIGURE 6-9
### GENERAL-REVENUE SHARE: 2011 TECHNOLOGY
### VERSUS CURRENT MEDICARE EXPENDITURES

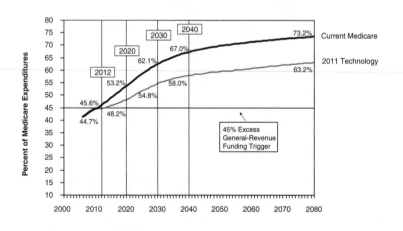

SOURCES: Authors' estimates and from Table III.A2. and Figure III.A1., *2006 Medicare Trustees Report* and Table VI.F4., *2006 Social Security Trustees Report*.

from that of Current Medicare. By 2020, however, the share of 2011 Technology Medicare is fully five percentage points smaller than Current Medicare. At the close of the seventy-five-year projection period, the general-revenue share of all Medicare expenditures is fully ten percentage points different.

## Conclusion

In this chapter we have estimated the financial impact of fixing the level of health-care technology that exists when a cohort reaches the Medicare age of eligibility. Here we fixed the technology for each eligible cohort separately and then fixed the technology at a specific date for all future cohorts. Neither reform, by itself, is sufficient to make Medicare solvent. Indeed, both result in a finding of "excess general-revenue funding," as defined in the 2003 MMA, within twenty-five years. One way to compare the two forms of fixing technology is to review their impact on the level of the transfer required at the close of the trustees' seventy-five-year projection period. As we have said before, this comparison is useful because, given the assumption by the trustees that at the close of this period health-care spending growth will be equal to the growth rate of per-capita GDP, the shares of general revenue required to fund Medicare will remain at the share estimated in the terminal year of the projection period.

In figure 6-10 (on the following page), we show the terminal-year share of federal nonentitlement revenues required to pay for the government's share of Medicare relative to Current Medicare. Allowing for health-care cost growth up to the time of retirement and then price-indexing thereafter, Retirement Technology Medicare produces a terminal-year transfer of about 81 percent that of Current Medicare. However, the much more aggressive reform of fixing technology at a fixed date and allowing only per-capita GDP growth to the year of retirement, 2011 Technology Medicare, has a much greater effect. For this reform, the terminal-year transfer is less than half that required by Current Medicare, but it will still require more than one-third of all federal nonentitlement revenues at the close of the seventy-five-year projection period.

FIGURE 6-10
TERMINAL-YEAR SHARE OF NONENTITLEMENT REVENUES: RETIREMENT
TECHNOLOGY VERSUS 2011 TECHNOLOGY MEDICARE
Relative to Current Medicare (percent)

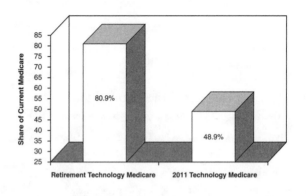

SOURCE: Authors' estimates.

The terminal values of the required transfers identify critical values in evaluating the reforms, but they do not reflect the aggregate debt of the system. Figure 6-11 shows the seventy-five-year unfunded liability for Current Medicare and each of the two technology-fixed reforms. Current Medicare has a $32.4 trillion unfunded liability. Retirement Technology Medicare reduces this debt by 22 percent, while 2011 Technology Medicare wipes out fully 40 percent of the seventy-five-year unfunded liability.

In figure 6-12, we show the seventy-five-year unfunded liability for each of the fixed-technology Medicare reforms relative to Current Medicare. While this figure is similar to figure 6-10, where we show required general-revenue transfers for each reform relative to the transfers that Current Medicare would require, the magnitudes of the relative reductions in unfunded liability are almost uniformly smaller than those in terminal-year transfers shown in figure 6-10. Because the trustees' current approach to projecting the long run assumes that by 2080, the growth of health-care expenditures will equal that of per-capita GDP, the terminal-year transfers as a share of general revenues approximate the long run.

FIGURE 6-11
SEVENTY-FIVE-YEAR UNFUNDED LIABILITY

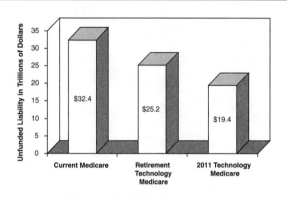

SOURCES: Authors' estimates and Table V.E2., *2006 Medicare Trustees Report.*

FIGURE 6-12
SEVENTY-FIVE-YEAR UNFUNDED LIABILITY RELATIVE TO CURRENT MEDICARE

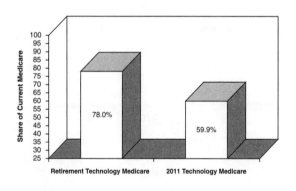

SOURCE: Authors' estimates.

Since the seventy-five-year unfunded liability is the present value of the required general-revenue transfers, its reduction depends greatly on when the reductions in funding take place. Not surprisingly, 2011

Technology Medicare, which results in the largest reduction in the transfer relative to Current Medicare at the close of the period, is also better than Retirement Technology Medicare in reducing the seventy-five-year unfunded liability.

# 7

# Scoring Medicare Reform III: Controlling First-Dollar Coverage

While the reforms considered in chapters 5 and 6 would transfer some part of the cost of Medicare to users—Commission Medicare—or a significant part to users—technology-fixing reforms—we evaluated them as if they had little or no effect on the level of expenditures. The reform discussed here—the elimination of first-dollar coverage—is designed to reduce the reliance of the program on general revenues and to affect the level of overall spending. The available evidence from the RAND Health Insurance Experiment suggests that the elimination of first-dollar coverage—that is, health-care coverage without a deductible amount—can have significant effects on the demand for health care, especially at the outpatient level.

## Controlling First-Dollar Coverage

There is general agreement that the prevalence of Medigap insurance among the Medicare population results in an increased level of health-care expenditures.[1] Medigap insurance is designed to cover the gaps in Medicare. From the perspective of pure insurance, Medicare does not cover the catastrophic costs associated with a long-lasting, expensive condition. It is natural for risk-averse individuals to desire to insure against very costly but very unlikely events. The catastrophic nature of Medigap is the culprit

---

1. See, for example, Frech (1999) for a discussion of the effect of Medigap coverage on Medicare spending and Shaviro (2004) for a discussion of the effectiveness of deductibles and copays in affecting the level of health-care consumption.

in producing higher spending, however. Medigap essentially removes all the deductibles and copays that are Medicare's primary cost-control mechanisms. Because over 85 percent of Medicare beneficiaries have some form of individual or employer-sponsored Medigap insurance or are covered by Medicaid, the Medicare population essentially has first-dollar coverage when it comes to health-care consumption.

An appropriate reform to control Medigap would include catastrophic coverage in Medicare and would prohibit the purchase of insurance that eliminates Medicare's deductibles and copays. One would expect that a prohibition of Medigap would not be necessary because the cost of coverage would exceed the deductibles, given adverse selection, and there would be little or no demand for the product at that price. Coupled with the elimination of Medigap, the extension and increase in coinsurance have been a common denominator in discussions of Medicare reform.

A benchmark for the relative effects of coinsurance rates and some level of no-first-dollar coverage on the level of medical expenditures can be estimated based on the results from the RAND Health Insurance Experiment (HIE). Manning et al. (1988) estimated that, relative to free care, a policy with 100 percent coinsurance after the first $1,000 would reduce hospital expenditures by 27.4 percent and all other expenditures, including acute, well, and chronic care, by 49.3 percent. The $1,000 deductible is in 1983 dollars. Adjusting this deductible using per-capita Medicare cost growth for Parts A and B produces a 2006-dollar equivalent of $4,642.

Individuals with Medigap insurance face the same prices—essentially zero—as those with free care in the RAND Experiment. Using data from the 1994 National Health Interview Survey (U.S. Department of Health and Human Services 1994), Christensen and Shinogle (1997) found evidence that beneficiaries with Medigap plans used 28 percent more services than those with no supplement. They also found that Medicare beneficiaries with employer-based supplements used 17 percent more services.[2] Medicare beneficiaries with no Medigap or employer-based supplements face the

---

2. Using data from the 1995 Medicare Current Beneficiary Surveys (MCBS; U.S. Department of Health and Human Services), we tested for adverse selection in the purchase of Medigap coverage by regressing Medigap coverage on health status along with other controls and found no systematic effects.

deductibles imposed in Parts A and B and the 20 percent Part B coinsurance rate, as well as the Part A coinsurance rate that comes into effect during hospital stays in excess of sixty days. Since the RAND Experiment results are confirmed by the Medigap study, we use them in our estimates of the cost of a no-first-dollar-coverage health-insurance alternative to Current Medicare.

To estimate the effects of no-first-dollar-coverage health insurance on Medicare spending, we use the simulation model output from the RAND Experiment presented in appendix G of Manning et al. Current Medicare with Medigap and Medicaid is essentially equivalent to the free care in the RAND Experiment. We estimate the effects of replacing current Medicare with a $5,000-deductible policy with no copays above the deductible, using the RAND Experiment results based on the $1,000 Maximum Dollar Expenditure (MDE) policy, with no copayments above the deductible. The difference between the simulated Medicare results and the results for our alternative plan as a percentage of simulated Medicare is our estimate of the expected percentage reduction for each category of expenditures. For purposes of this estimation, we assume that all current Medicare beneficiaries buy Medigap coverage.[3]

Specifically, we assume that in accordance with the RAND Experiment's results for the $1,000 MDE policy, hospitalization expenditures will be equal to 72.62 percent, and Parts B and D expenditures equal to 50.67 percent, of a free-care policy.[4] In addition, we assume the deductible will rise at the rate of per-capita Medicare expenditures.

We assume that the reform begins immediately, and that its full effect is immediate; gradual adjustment to the reform would make the initial impact smaller but would not affect the long run.

Figure 7-1 (on the following page) shows the transfers required to fund No-First-Dollar Medicare and Current Medicare as shares of federal non-entitlement revenues. Because we have assumed that the full effect of the reform is immediate, the general-revenue transfer is reduced by more than

---

3. Those who do not buy coverage are at the lower end of health-care usage, so the effect of this assumption on the total saving is minimal.

4. Our estimates are based on changes in expected spending between the free-care and $1,000 MDE policy. Confidence limits are provided in the RAND Experiment results, but for our purposes only the average effect is used.

FIGURE 7-1
REQUIRED TRANSFERS: NO-FIRST-DOLLAR MEDICARE
Percent Federal Nonentitlement Revenues

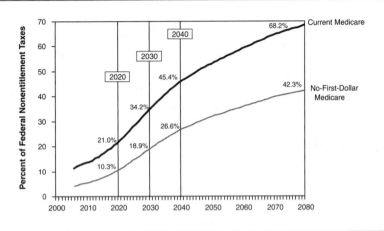

SOURCE: Authors' estimates.
NOTE: Federal nonentitlement taxes are estimated to be 11.8 percent of GDP, the twenty-five-year average.

60 percent from its current level of 11.2 percent of nonentitlement revenues to 4.1 percent. While the reduction over the entire seventy-five-year trustees' projection period remains very significant, the percentage reduction is less impressive than the initial reduction in general-revenue transfers.

No-First-Dollar Medicare significantly reduces the system's long-run funding requirements, but this benefit reform alone can only go so far toward solving Medicare's shortfalls. In less than fifteen years, the level of transfers required is almost as high as the current level required for Current Medicare, 10.3 percent versus 11.2 percent. By 2030, a transfer of almost 19 percent of federal nonentitlement revenues to Medicare will be required, and by 2040 the transfer will need to be more than 25 percent. At the close of the seventy-five-year projection period, No-First-Dollar Medicare would require a transfer of more than 42 percent of all nonentitlement revenues to Medicare. While this terminal-year transfer is almost 40 percent smaller than Current Medicare would require, nonentitlement revenues would have to rise or nonentitlement expenditures would have to be reduced significantly to make it.

Moving to No-First-Dollar Medicare reduces Medicare's reliance on general revenues, but it does not eliminate the need for significant future transfers. In particular, the MMA requirement of a finding of "excess general-revenue transfer" would remain an issue. For Current Medicare, the 45 percent level triggering the warning to the president was reached for the first time in 2006. Given the current Medicare trustees' projections, the warning can be expected to be repeated in 2007.

The projections of general-revenue share for both Current Medicare and No-First-Dollar Medicare are depicted in figure 7-2, which shows that while No-First-Dollar Medicare implies a significantly smaller initial general-revenue share—roughly half of Current Medicare—in less than twenty years (2024), it still reaches the critical 45 percent required for the determination of excess general-revenue funding. The initial improvement is a result of our assuming that the reduction in expenditures resulting from the reform is immediate. Further, we have assumed that the expenditure reductions are limited to level-of-expenditure effects, and that they have no effect on the rate of growth in Medicare spending. This analysis indicates that the

FIGURE 7-2

**GENERAL-REVENUE SHARE: NO-FIRST-DOLLAR VERSUS CURRENT MEDICARE EXPENDITURES**

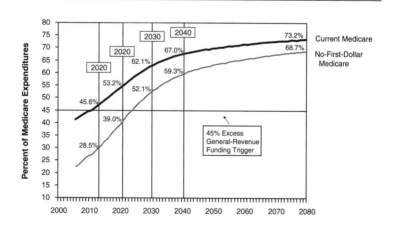

SOURCES: Authors' estimates and Table III.A2. and Figure III.A1., *2006 Medicare Trustees Report* and Table VI.F4., *2006 Social Security Trustees Report*.

solution to creating a Medicare that will be financially sound cannot be found in the elimination of first-dollar coverage alone unless this institutional change also provokes slower per-capita spending growth.

## Conclusion

The reform perhaps most likely to reduce the level of expenditures projected by the trustees is the elimination of first-dollar coverage. It also has the greatest potential to reduce per-capita spending growth. Once again, it is clear that no reform by itself is sufficient to make Medicare solvent unless it provokes lower spending growth than is projected. We do not attempt to estimate reductions in per-capita expenditure growth rates for any of the reforms we consider, though such reductions would be expected, particularly with this reform. Figure 7-3 shows the federal nonentitlement revenues required to pay the government's share of No-First-Dollar Medicare and Current Medicare in the final projection year. Even a very effective cost-reducing reform, such as the movement to No-First-Dollar Medicare, still requires more than one-third of all nonentitlement revenues at the close of the projection period.

FIGURE 7-3

TERMINAL-YEAR SHARE OF NONENTITLEMENT REVENUES:
NO-FIRST-DOLLAR AND CURRENT MEDICARE

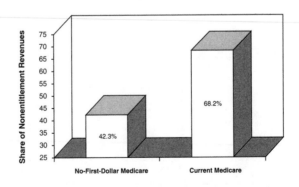

SOURCE: Authors' estimates.

As with the other reforms examined thus far, we now consider the degree to which No-First-Dollar Medicare reduces the present value of the seventy-five-year unfunded obligation. The unfunded liabilities for No-First-Dollar Medicare and Current Medicare are given in figure 7-4. The movement to No-First-Dollar Medicare wipes out over 40 percent of Current Medicare's $32.4 trillion–dollar liability.

FIGURE 7-4
SEVENTY-FIVE-YEAR UNFUNDED LIABILITY

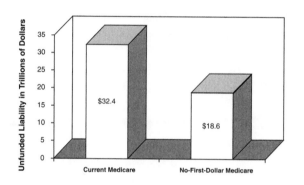

SOURCES: Authors' estimates and table V.E2., *2006 Medicare Trustees Report.*

Imposing No-First-Dollar Medicare would result in this large reduction because it is assumed to have an immediate and lasting impact on the level of health-care expenditures. Further, the liability is a present-value calculation. Thus, the fact that No-First-Dollar Medicare is assumed to have an immediate and significant effect on Medicare expenditures magnifies the early-year benefit of No-First-Dollar relative to Current Medicare. Further, it should be reiterated that these estimates summarize the effect of the reform on the federal government's ledger. Retirees will be responsible for the higher deductible, and their health-care consumption will be less than the amount currently projected.

In the next chapter we look at the last in our set of Medicare reforms, Means-Tested Medicare. While the 2003 MMA introduced a limited form of means-testing for Medicare Part B, the level of income required before means-testing has any bite is high enough that the long-run effect on premium revenues is projected to be limited. The form of means-testing we analyze is more aggressive and applies to all Medicare, not just Part B.

# 8

# Scoring Medicare Reform IV:
# Means-Tested Medicare

The reforms considered up to this point transfer some part of the cost of Medicare to users in general. In contrast, the reform discussed in this chapter limits the cost transfer, in the form of reduced benefits, to those elderly people with the highest incomes. Increasing the share of health-care expenditures that are covered by beneficiaries has the potential to alter the incentives of those who are most affected. Indeed, Pauly (1999a) argues that, in addition to transferring some of the cost of Medicare to users, the significant increase in premiums associated with aggressive means-testing could result in individuals declining coverage and becoming more price-conscious. As in the previous chapter, we ignore the possible incentive effects facing higher-income beneficiaries.

## Means-Tested Medicare

Unlike Social Security, which is paid for exclusively by dedicated payroll taxes, Medicare has been paid for partially by payroll taxes (Part A) and partially by a combination of premiums and general-revenue transfers (Parts B and D). One way to limit the extent of general-revenue transfers as the source of Medicare funding is to means-test either the level of benefits provided or the premium that beneficiaries pay for these benefits. Essentially, means-testing is a way of increasing the share of the Medicare financing burden that is borne by the higher-income elderly. This reform has the potential, if the means-testing is aggressive enough, to affect the participation of the elderly, and perhaps their level of health-care expenditures.

However, because we have no information on the private insurance market that would exist in the presence of a large set of elderly who opted out of Medicare, we assume in our analysis that total spending by the elderly population will be as projected in the *2006 Medicare Trustees Report*.

In 2003, the MMA introduced limited means-testing in the determination of Medicare Part B premiums. Here we go well beyond the MMA, in that in addition to increasing the premiums for those elderly with greater means, we reduce the level of coverage as a beneficiary's income rises, as suggested by Pauly (1999a and 1999b). Pauly argues that such a move increases efficiency in that, at least for higher-income seniors, medical decisions will be made with the real cost in mind rather than a zero or minimal individual cost relative to other real resource costs. To the extent that such a change reduces the immediate burden on current workers through a reduced payroll tax, it will have positive labor-supply effects. However, to the extent that an increase in work effort and earnings when one is young simply means that one will be required to relinquish the wealth after retirement as a result of reduced Medicare benefits, an individual can be expected to reduce his or her work effort.

## Methodology

We structure this reform in a way similar to the Part B subsidy-reduction provisions of the 2003 MMA. Rather than basing the reductions on fixed ranges of adjusted gross income that are updated annually for inflation, we relate the subsidy to the definition of poverty according to federal definitions. We use the Federal Reserve's 2004 Survey of Consumer Finances (SCF; U.S. Federal Reserve Board 2004) to identify the income distribution in 2003 for individuals ages sixty-five and over. These data are used to create age-group-specific means-testing factors, which are then applied to average spending at each age.[1]

---

1. All income estimates in the SCF are weighted based on the revised weights. There are nine age categories: one for each age, sixty-five to sixty-nine, for a total of five single-age categories; three five-year age categories for ages seventy to seventy-four, seventy-five to seventy-nine, and eighty to eighty-four; and a final category for ages eighty-five and over. Other surveys besides the SCF could be used to identify the distribution of income among the elderly, like the Current Population Survey, the Consumer Expenditure Survey, or the Health and Retirement Study.

To estimate the factors, we begin by identifying the poverty threshold for each household in the SCF. The families' total incomes in 2003, which for retiree households are basically adjusted gross income, are compared to the poverty threshold for the household. To give the reform structure, we identify seven income categories relative to the poverty levels for the retiree's household. For each age group, the percentages of individuals who fall into the seven income categories are determined.

The income categories, along with the means-testing factors, are given in table 8-1. For these estimates of the impact of means-testing on Medicare expenditures, the age-specific income distribution that existed in 2003 is used to calculate the effects of means-testing in all future years. Other income thresholds or means-testing factors could have been employed for this exercise, but these produce an outcome that is comparable to the previous reforms we have discussed.

Since with Current Medicare the poor, however defined, are exempt from premiums for Parts B and D, we retain this low-income subsidy in our estimates. Thus, as indicated in the table, individuals in households at or below 150 percent of the poverty threshold continue to receive 100 percent of the projected age-specific transfer. As household incomes rise, however, the average transfer falls, such that individuals in a household with income at or above nine times the poverty threshold receive a transfer of only 20 percent of projected age-specific expenditures.

To illustrate the levels of income involved, the poverty threshold in 2003 for a household of two in which the householder was sixty-five or older was $11,333. Thus, individuals in households of two with income of $17,000 ($11,333*1.5) or less in 2003 would receive 100 percent of the projected age-specific Medicare transfer. At the upper income levels, individuals in households of two with incomes of $102,000 or more would receive a transfer equal to 20 percent of the age-specific amount. Between these two thresholds, the transfer declines from 100 percent to 20 percent. By way of comparison, means-testing in the 2003 MMA began at $80,000 for an individual and $160,000 for a couple. Thus, our means-testing formula is considerably more aggressive than MMA's and also covers all of Medicare, not just Part B.

The effects of this particular form of means-testing on the Medicare benefits can be illustrated by considering the case of individuals who are sixty-seven years old. Table 8-2 identifies the distribution of individuals across the

TABLE 8-1

INCOME THRESHOLDS AND TRANSFER PERCENTAGES: MEANS-TESTING EXAMPLE

| Income Category | Household Income Compared to Poverty Threshold | Transfer as a Percent of Projected Age-Specific Spending |
|:---:|:---:|:---:|
| 1 | income ≤ poverty threshold • 1.5 | 100.00 |
| 2 | poverty threshold • 1.5 < income ≤ poverty threshold • 3.0 | 86.67 |
| 3 | poverty threshold • 3.0 < income ≤ poverty threshold • 4.5 | 73.33 |
| 4 | poverty threshold • 4.5 < income ≤ poverty threshold • 6.0 | 60.00 |
| 5 | poverty threshold • 6.0 < income ≤ poverty threshold • 7.5 | 46.67 |
| 6 | poverty threshold • 7.5 < income ≤ poverty threshold • 9.0 | 33.33 |
| 7 | poverty threshold • 9.0 < income | 20.00 |

SOURCE: Authors' estimates from the 2004 Survey of Consumer Finances, United States Federal Reserve.

seven income categories from the 2004 SCF. Almost one-quarter of the sixty-seven-year-olds would receive 100 percent of their projected Medicare benefits, while about 12 percent would fall in the topmost income category and receive only the 20 percent transfer. The overall weighted average applied to average spending is the sum of the products of the percentage in each category and the income-based transfer percentage. For those sixty-seven years old, the weighted average factor applied to spending is 67.53 percent. The means-testing factor generally rises with age with the oldest group, those eighty-five and older, to 84.85 percent. This means that, on average, the Medicare transfer to individuals in this age group will equal about 85 percent of the scheduled benefits, based on the means-adjusting methodology we have outlined.

**Effect of Means-Adjusting on Aggregate Medicare Spending**

Figure 8-1 compares the transfers required to fund Means-Tested Medicare versus Current Medicare in terms of federal nonentitlement revenues. Means-Tested Medicare improves the long-run outlook more than

TABLE 8-2

**MEANS-TESTING FACTOR EXAMPLE FOR INDIVIDUALS
SIXTY-SEVEN YEARS OF AGE IN 2003**

| Income Category | Percentage in Category | Projected Age Specific Spending | Transfer as a Percent of Means-Testing Factor |
|---|---|---|---|
| 1 | 23.12 | 100.00 | 23.12 |
| 2 | 11.07 | 86.67 | 9.81 |
| 3 | 19.16 | 73.33 | 14.05 |
| 4 | 21.38 | 60.00 | 12.83 |
| 5 | 7.05 | 46.67 | 3.29 |
| 6 | 5.85 | 33.33 | 1.95 |
| 7 | 12.36 | 20.00 | 2.47 |
| Total | 100.00% | | 67.53% |

SOURCE: Authors' estimates from the 2004 Survey of Consumer Finances, United States Federal Reserve.

FIGURE 8-1

**REQUIRED TRANSFERS: MEANS-TESTED VERSUS CURRENT MEDICARE
Percent Federal Nonentitlement Revenues**

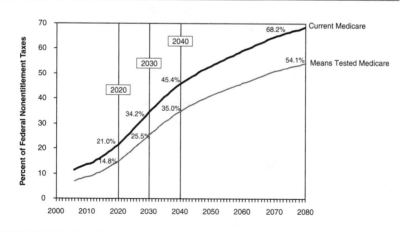

SOURCE: Authors' estimates.
NOTE: Federal nonentitlement taxes are estimated to be 11.8 percent of GDP, the twenty-five-year average.

Commission Medicare or Retirement Technology Medicare, but, like the others, it falls short of being a total solution to funding shortfalls. With this reform, Medicare will need transfers of almost 15 percent of nonentitlement revenues in less than fifteen years, of more than 25 percent by 2030, and of 35 percent in 2040. By 2080, Means-Tested Medicare would require a transfer of more than 54 percent of all nonentitlement revenues.

Our other comparison of Means-Tested Medicare and Current Medicare based on general-revenue transfers as a percentage of total spending is given in figure 8-2. While the figure shows that the movement to this form of Means-Tested Medicare implies a significantly smaller initial share of general revenue—about 80 percent of the burden of Current Medicare—it still reaches the critical 45 percent threshold only seven years later. The initial improvement is a result of our assuming that the reduction in Medicare-paid expenditures resulting from the reform is immediate. Again, much as we concluded in our analyses of the other reforms, Means-Tested Medicare would have to be combined with other reforms to bring the system's cost and revenues together in the long run.

FIGURE 8-2
**GENERAL-REVENUE SHARE: MEANS-TESTED
VERSUS CURRENT MEDICARE EXPENDITURES**

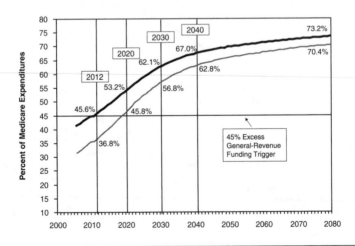

SOURCES: Authors' estimates and table III.A2. and Figure III.A1., *2006 Medicare Trustees Report* and Table VI.F4., *2006 Social Security Trustees Report.*

## Conclusion

Aggressive means-testing would seem to have the potential to reduce significantly the dependence of Medicare on general revenues. However, as estimated, its effect is muted given the structure we adopted and its application to the distribution of income among the elderly. The terminal-year share of nonentitlement revenues required to pay for the government's share of Means-Tested Medicare relative to Current Medicare is shown in figure 8-3. While means-testing makes a significant reduction in the share of nonentitlement revenues required, the level of the transfer is still over half of all such revenues.

FIGURE 8-3
TERMINAL-YEAR SHARE OF NONENTITLEMENT REVENUES:
MEANS-TESTED VERSUS CURRENT MEDICARE

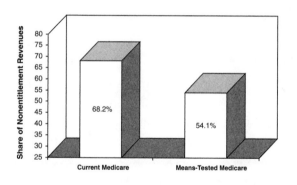

SOURCE: Authors' estimates.

Looking at how the trustees summarize the impact of Medicare for the current and future taxpayer in terms of the seventy-five-year unfunded liability, we show these amounts in figure 8-4 for Current Medicare and Means-Tested Medicare. Current Medicare has a $32.4 trillion unfunded liability. Means-Tested Medicare reduces this figure by $7.7 trillion, to $24.7 trillion. The way we score Means-Tested and No-First-Dollar Medicare imposes the reforms immediately, and the almost 24 percent

FIGURE 8-4
SEVENTY-FIVE-YEAR UNFUNDED LIABILITY

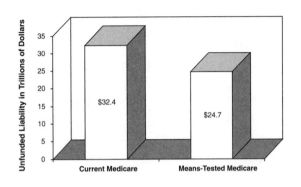

SOURCES: Authors' estimates and Table V.E2., *2006 Medicare Trustees Report.*

reduction in the seventy-five-year unfunded liability is at least partially due to this assumption.

We also note here that in our scoring of Means-Tested Medicare, we have assumed that even the highest-income seniors remain in the system, simply replacing the 80 percent of Medicare benefits they are denied with their own insurance. But, again, as Pauly (1999a) has argued, it is likely that the low benefits offered the high-income seniors will induce them to leave the system. Thus, there is the potential for a significant incentive effect which would reduce overall health-care usage by seniors, although its effect on Medicare financing is uncertain. To the extent that high-income seniors are also healthier, they would have been lower users of the system. The average subsidy of 20 percent of per-capita age-adjusted expenditures received by the highest-income seniors would prompt the healthiest to leave the system, taking their premium contributions with them.

In the following chapter, we summarize the findings of all of the reform evaluations. We summarize the effects of the reforms from the vantage point of the Medicare system, cognizant of the fact that any cost savings to Medicare, or taxpayers, imply higher costs for retirees. Thus, we ignore possibly important components of the postreform world: First, all the reforms we consider are essentially benefit reductions. This has implications for preretirement consumption decisions, as workers must prepare to pay for more of their retirement health care than the current system promises but perhaps cannot deliver. Second, we assume that the reforms, other than the no-first-dollar reform, leave desired health-care consumption by seniors unchanged. How seniors pay for the difference between covered and noncovered expenditures may affect incentives and, ultimately, desired expenditures, and the growth rate in total per-capita spending.

# 9

# What Can Reform Accomplish?
# The Medicare Reform Scores

All of the reforms considered in chapters 5–8 will transfer some part of the cost of Current Medicare to users. In our scoring of these proposals, we have evaluated them from the point of view of the Centers for Medicaid and Medicare Services (CMS) and not the beneficiaries. In addition, except for the no-first-dollar reform, we ignored the impact the reforms might have on the incentives of beneficiaries and therefore on the level of expenditures as projected by the Medicare trustees.

While the reforms have all appeared in one form or another in other places, in order to estimate their imposition a formal structure for each had to be assumed. The reform recommended by the National Bipartisan Commission on the Future of Medicare was scored in chapter 5. In the time that has passed since the 1999 final report of the commission, Medicare has changed and become more like the program the commission envisioned. In our scoring of Commission Medicare we assumed, for reasons outlined in chapter 5, that the only significant difference between it and Current Medicare was the adoption of Social Security's full retirement age as the Medicare age of eligibility.

Given this recommendation, it was natural to consider a reform that combined the Social Security initial-benefit calculation with the price-indexing inherent in Social Security's benefit structure. We denoted this second reform as Retirement Technology Medicare. In this reform, the age-benefit structure in existence in the year a beneficiary retires, as derived from the *2006 Medicare Trustees Reports*, is subsequently adjusted during his or her retirement by real economy-wide price-level changes, as is done with Social Security benefits. Thus, the initial-benefit profile is adjusted for the health-care expenditure growth to the year of retirement, but the age-benefit profile remains fixed in real terms at the levels that existed the year of retirement. Initial benefits are thereby health-care cost-indexed, but subsequent benefit levels are indexed to per-capita GDP growth.

An extension of this reform is based on an aspect of many Social Security reform proposals, namely, fixing the retirement benefit at a point in time and only price-indexing the benefit to be received by future cohorts. Essentially, this reform, referred to as "price-indexing," fixes the real purchasing power of retirement benefits for all future retirees. Such a reform requires future retirees to provide for themselves all levels of expenditures beyond this base level. We did not go this far in slowing benefit growth in the reform we priced. Rather, we allowed the beginning age-benefit profile, defined as the age-benefit profile that exists in 2011, to rise by per-capita GDP growth, which historically has been considerably lower than health-care cost growth but considerably above the zero real growth assumed if the fixed-date age-benefit profile were only price-indexed. This reform is the more generous counterpart to the Social Security reform that fixes the benefit structure as of a particular date and only price-indexes thereafter, as opposed to the current policy of wage-indexing the beginning benefit level for future cohorts.

The third reform is based on the evidence that third-party payments in health care have led to consumption in excess of what would exist if consumers actually paid marginal costs. The reform we analyzed eliminates first-dollar-coverage through a universal Medicare policy that had a $5,000 deductible, with zero copay above the deductible. We used the results of the RAND Health Insurance Experiment as a basis for estimating the impact of No-First-Dollar Medicare on the level of expenditures for the various parts of Medicare.

The fourth and final reform considered was a relatively aggressive means-testing of Medicare benefits. Here we combined all parts of Medicare and took away current benefits according to the income level of the elderly. We estimated the cost-saving to Medicare using data on the elderly income distribution and a benefit-reduction schedule that provides 100 percent of benefits to individuals in families at or below 150 percent of poverty level, and that gradually reduces benefits as income rises, so that only 20 percent of current benefits are available for individuals living in families with the highest income levels.

Given the wide variety of suggestions for reforming Medicare, it is surprising so few estimates have been offered of the contribution that any one
of them, if enacted, would make toward solving Medicare's looming financial crisis. None of the reforms we evaluated is sufficient, by itself, to make
Medicare solvent. Indeed, every one results in a finding of "excess general-
revenue funding," as defined in the 2003 MMA, within twenty-five years.

One way to compare the set of reforms we have scored is to review their
impact on the level of the transfer required at the close of the trustees'
seventy-five-year projection period. This comparison is useful because the
trustees assume that by the end of this period health-care spending growth
will be equal to the growth rate of per-capita GDP. Consequently, the shares
of general revenue required to fund Medicare will remain at the share estimated for 2080, the terminal year of the period.

Table 9-1 shows the share of federal nonentitlement revenues required
to pay for the government's share of Medicare for all reforms for the years
2020, 2030, 2040, and 2080, the last year of the seventy-five-year projection period. The reforms are listed in the table according to their terminal
required transfer. Given the trustees' assumption that by the year 2080 the
growth of per-capita health-care expenditures will match the growth in per-
capita GDP, the terminal-year transfers as a share of nonentitlement revenues approximate the long-run transfer levels. They range from Current
Medicare's transfer of 68.42 percent to 2011 Technology Medicare's transfer of 35.93 percent of projected nonentitlement revenues.

TABLE 9-1

REQUIRED SHARE PERCENTAGES OF FEDERAL NONENTITLEMENT REVENUES

| Year | Current Medicare | Commission Medicare | Retirement Technology Medicare | Means-Tested Medicare | No-First-Dollar Medicare | 2011 Technology Medicare |
|------|------------------|---------------------|--------------------------------|-----------------------|--------------------------|--------------------------|
| 2020 | 21.14 | 18.01 | 16.97 | 14.94 | 8.00 | 17.34 |
| 2030 | 34.31 | 30.06 | 25.87 | 25.64 | 16.01 | 24.82 |
| 2040 | 45.59 | 40.26 | 33.37 | 35.23 | 23.10 | 29.22 |
| 2080 | 68.42 | 60.85 | 55.03 | 54.44 | 37.62 | 35.93 |

SOURCE: Authors' estimates.

Importantly, none of the reforms we scored would prevent the system from being subject to the finding of "excess general-revenue funding." Figure 9-1 shows the level of the terminal-year general-revenue funding share of total Medicare expenditures. Note at the top of each column the year that each Medicare reaches the critical 45 percent level of general-revenue funding. Not surprisingly, Current Medicare reaches the critical level before any of the reformed systems, and its terminal level of general-revenue support is the greatest.

The reform that performs the best in terms of terminal general-revenue funding—fixing the technology at 2011—reaches the critical level just two years later than Current Medicare. This seeming anomaly is a result of the fact that the initial year of the reform was 2011, when the general-revenue transfer was almost at 45 percent. The reform that performs almost as well as 2011 Technology Medicare, No-First-Dollar Medicare, reaches the critical level latest, in 2024—twelve years later than Current Medicare. Again, the reason is transparent. For No-First-Dollar Medicare, the full effects are assumed to occur immediately and continue throughout the projection period.

FIGURE 9-1

**REQUIRED 2080 GENERAL-REVENUE TRANSFER AND YEAR OF "EXCESS-GENERAL REVENUE FUNDING"**

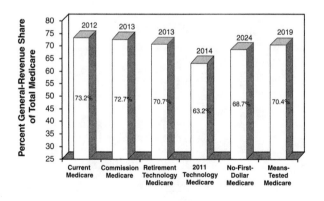

SOURCES: Authors' estimates and from Table III.A2. and Figure III.A1., *2006 Medicare Trustees Report* and Table VI.F4., *2006 Social Security Trustees Report*.

In terms of financing the deficits inherent in Current Medicare and all of the scored reforms, the contribution of any of the reforms to the seventy-five-year unfunded Medicare debt is every bit as important as the level of general-revenue transfers. Figure 9-2 shows the seventy-five-year unfunded liabilities for Current Medicare and each reform. Current Medicare has a $32.4 trillion unfunded liability. Commission Medicare, which brings the age of eligibility for Medicare in line with the full retirement age of Social Security, pays off just under $2 trillion of this liability. Means-Tested Medicare and Retirement Technology Medicare give us, respectively, reductions of $7.2 and $7.7 trillion.

We get the most from reform programs that aggressively reduce the share of benefits paid by the government. The first of these—fixing the benefits at a certain date and letting future beneficiaries pay for all technology and cost increases above the growth of per-capita GDP—wipes out 40 percent of Current Medicare's seventy-five-year unfunded liability. However, we get the most from a reform that not only changes who pays, but affects the level of expenditures as well. No-First-Dollar Medicare wipes out just under 43 percent of Current Medicare's seventy-five-year liability.

FIGURE 9-2

SEVENTY-FIVE-YEAR UNFUNDED LIABILITY

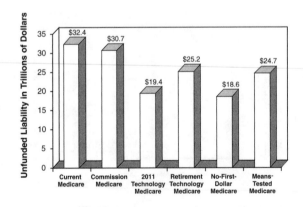

SOURCES: Authors' estimates and Table V.E2., *2006 Medicare Trustees Report*.

With this review of the reforms we have set the stage for a discussion of changing the way that Medicare is financed. Specifically, we introduce the idea of moving from the generational-transfer method of financing to cohort-based prepayment of future health-care consumption. Given the scale of the projected funding requirements, Medicare cannot and will not remain in its current form. To the extent that changes in the program involve benefit reductions, they imply that workers will have to prepare for retirement by prepayment for some of their retirement health care. The approach we take in the following chapter estimates the level of contributions that would be required to fund fully Current Medicare and each of the reformed systems evaluated in chapters 5–8.

# 10

# The Fundamentals of Prepaying Medicare

In a previous book (Rettenmaier and Saving 2000) we proposed prepaying retirement health insurance. Prepaying retirement health insurance is similar to prepaying other retirement consumption and can be accomplished individually or corporately. Individuals can either set aside funds in retirement health-insurance accounts that cover health-care spending in their old age, just as they save for other retirement consumption by setting aside funds in their 401(k) plans, or they can contribute to a retirement health-pension fund similar to defined-benefit pension funds sponsored by employers and unions.

Over the past several years, we have recommended individualized prepayment of a particular form. For the purpose of this chapter, however, we are not necessarily concerned about the particular vehicle used to prepay Medicare but, rather, are interested in illustrating the general concept of prepayment. We will begin with a discussion of how prepayment will work, review its costs, and, finally, address some common concerns. Along the way we will identify which generations are net beneficiaries of Medicare in its current form and which are net payers into the program. The following chapter will then address the transition from the current generational-transfer system to prepaid retirement health insurance.

## The Idea

In its simplest form, prepaid retirement health insurance involves paying an annual premium throughout one's preretirement years that secures coverage of health-care expenses during retirement. The insurance contract begins when a worker is young and continues to death. Claims are contingent upon survival to retirement age, and then upon the event of adverse health shocks during retirement. In these ways, the insurance resembles Medicare's Part A Hospital Insurance (HI). HI payroll taxes are similar to the premiums we have in mind, and the claims on Part A are contingent upon reaching retirement age and on experiencing adverse health shocks. The prepaid program can also be universal in participation through mandatory contributions, just as HI tax payments are mandatory.

The health-insurance coverage in a prepaid system can be identical across individuals in retirement, just as Medicare is now. We will discuss the pros and cons of universal participation and identical coverage in a later chapter, but for now those issues can be tabled as we identify a basic pre-payment mechanism. The difference between the current transfer payment financing arrangement and the one we outline is that the premiums in the prepaid system are reserved in savings, or claims on capital, until retirement. Ownership rests with individuals rather than the discretion of some future Congress to honor the current system's commitments.

While chapters 5–8 scored in detail several reforms that would redefine Medicare's coverage and/or commitments to retirees, prepayment is a separate reform that would redefine how Medicare is financed. Having considered how the above reforms would affect Medicare's coverage and commitments, why should we go one step further and consider prepayment?

As we saw in the previous chapters, even a substantial reform that reduces Medicare's commitments to retirees in the future would still require revenues from taxpayers well above current funding levels. But Medicare is not the only federal program projected to make increasing demands on general revenues. Medicaid spending will also grow in future years for the dual-eligible within the retired population. More importantly, Social Security's loans to the rest of the federal government since 1983, now embodied in the Social Security Trust Fund, will have to be paid off when Social Security surpluses end and deficits begin in 2017. Together, the federal programs currently funding elderly consumption will produce significantly higher taxes within the next twenty years without reform. Prepaying retirement consumption can soften the blow on future taxpayers and has several other advantages, as well.

First, prepayment can have significant effects on the generational burden of financing Medicare. Future taxpayers will have a lower tax burden if members of the current working generation prepay, partially or entirely, their retirement health care. Conceptually, prepayment, at least in the case of Social Security, has had a difficult time politically because it may appear to benefit only future taxpayers while imposing a clear burden on current workers. Real prepayment requires current workers to set aside additional resources for the future, resulting in their consuming less today.

However, suppose one of the likely alternatives we have already discussed is adopted. Each of these reforms reduces benefits for future retirees from their currently projected levels. These retirees, who are today's workers, will then be required to pay much higher premiums, accept scaled-back coverage relative to scheduled coverage, or pay for more of their health care through higher copayments and deductibles. In any of these cases, it is the subsequent generation of taxpayers whose burden is reduced relative to the scheduled burden, thus achieving the same objective as prepayment. If these reductions are unanticipated, the burden of the reform is borne when today's workers are retirees and have substantially reduced abilities to adjust to the reduced transfer. So prepayment allows current workers, who are tomorrow's retirees, to anticipate the likely reductions in benefits relative to projected benefits while they are still in the labor force and have the ability to adjust.

Prepaying Medicare can also result in higher national saving than does the current generational-transfer financing arrangement. While the degree to which the current transfer-payment financing of Medicare or Social Security has reduced national saving is debatable, it is difficult to make the case that these programs have brought about no reduction. Medicare and Social Security transfer payments substitute for saving during the years of work. To the extent that prepayment of future Medicare results in an increased national saving rate, it will provide for a greater capital stock, resulting in a higher national income that will enhance the welfare of future generations.

## The Cost of Prepaying Medicare

We begin our analysis of the cost of prepaying Medicare by estimating the contribution rates as a percentage of lifetime earnings sufficient to pay for a cohort's expected health-care spending in retirement. For now, assume that contributions are held in a single community account for all members of a birth cohort. The account can be thought of as a retirement health-insurance pension plan, but rather than paying out defined benefits, it pays for an annual health-insurance premium.

To make the exercise more concrete, consider the case of individuals born in 1975, who were thirty-one years of age in 2006. Data on their earnings, expected Medicare benefits, and population counts or survival rates, as well as a rate of return that will be earned on the assets held in savings, are required for the calculation of a contribution rate. The contribution rate can be thought of as a fixed percentage of taxable earnings deposited in the community account.

Figure 10-1 (on the following page) presents the projected average earnings and current Medicare spending profiles by age for this birth year in constant 2006 dollars.[1] The contribution rate, or percentage of lifetime average earnings that is adequate to prepay scheduled benefits, is contingent on the discount rate we choose and the way in which we weight the earnings and benefits at each age. The implications of differing discount rates and weights are examined below.

Two real discount rates are used in the following examples. The lower rate of 2.9 percent is chosen to reflect the real government bond rate assumed in the *2006 Medicare Trustees Report*. It reflects the long-run opportunity cost of funds for the government and is appropriate for budgetary evaluations. The higher rate of 5.2 percent is consistent with the long-run real rate of return on a portfolio consisting of 60 percent equities and 40 percent bonds. It reflects individuals' opportunity costs.

In a closed economy, the contribution rate required to pay for the future benefits of a birth cohort would depend only on the income and mortality of the cohort. However, in an open economy, new entrants into the cohort must be taken into account. We must decide how to treat them in terms of the contribution rate they must pay for the benefits promised, or the benefits they are promised for the fixed-cohort contribution rate.

---

1. The Medicare spending profiles are again derived from the Continuous Medicare History Sample (CMHS; U.S. Department of Health and Human Services 2004) as discussed in chapter 6. The earnings data are based on average earners, computed using the method described in U.S. Social Security Administration (2005). The population data were provided by the Office of the Actuary, and the mortality data are from Bell and Miller (2005).

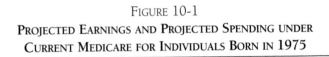

FIGURE 10-1

PROJECTED EARNINGS AND PROJECTED SPENDING UNDER
CURRENT MEDICARE FOR INDIVIDUALS BORN IN 1975

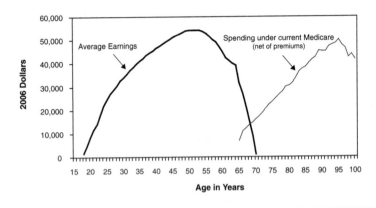

SOURCES: Authors' estimates based on earnings' scaling factors in U.S. Social Security Administration (2005) and from the Continuous Medicare History Sample.

To show the extent of this problem, we indicate in figure 10-2 the effect of immigration on the population of a birth cohort, using the population of individuals born in 1975. The two series in the figure are indexed to the population of the 1975 birth cohort at age eighteen—that is, its population at age eighteen is assumed to be one hundred. The population index, the upper line in the figure, shows the effects of immigration as the count of individuals born in 1975 actually grows and peaks at the age of forty-four, when the population is 17 percent larger than it was at eighteen. Based on Social Security Administration estimates, the number of individuals in the United States who were born in 1975 grows from just over 3.5 million when the cohort members are eighteen years of age, in 1993, to over 4.1 million when the cohort members are forty-four years of age, in 2019.

In contrast to these estimates based on Social Security Administration population projections, the survival function, also from the Social Security Administration, for this birth year—the lower line in the figure—suggests that 97 percent of the original members will survive to the age of forty-four. Thus, for this birth cohort by forty-four years of age, immigration has added 21 percent to the population that started out at the age of eighteen. Because of immigration, the total number of individuals in a given birth

FIGURE 10-2
POPULATION SURVIVAL INDEXED TO AGE EIGHTEEN
FOR INDIVIDUALS BORN IN 1975

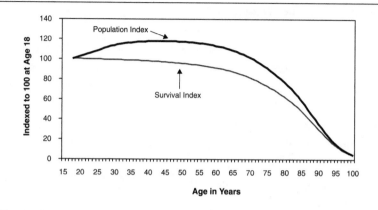

SOURCES: Authors' estimates from Social Security Administration population counts and life tables from Bell and Miller (2005).

cohort, beginning at eighteen years of age, rises, on average, until they are in their mid-forties.

If we require the contribution rate and benefits promised to be common for all members of a cohort, then the late arrivals are subsidized by those in the cohort at age eighteen. We refer to this estimated contribution rate as being population-weighted. The earnings and benefits for a given cohort are multiplied by its population at each age, to arrive at total earnings and total spending at each age. The fixed contribution rate, which will prepay benefits for all those in any given birth year, is simply the ratio of the aggregate discounted values of benefits to earnings, and is independent of country of birth. Thus, population weighting allows new entrants to the cohort to pay the same contribution rate and receive the same benefits as individuals who have contributed throughout their lives.[2]

---

2. While the new entrants will contribute to the community investment pool, individuals who contribute over their entire lifetimes actually subsidize later entrants and face higher contribution rates than they would with a pure insurance contract based only on survival rates.

As an alternative, the required contributions can be based on the date of entry into the cohort using the mortality tables. In this approach, which we shall hereafter refer to as mortality weighting, later entrants pay greater contribution rates determined in the same way as annuities. Thus, new entrants to such a contract would have to buy in at an actuarially adjusted higher contribution rate, or else would receive a lower benefit at retirement.

When the contribution rates for this birth year are calculated using the government bond rate of 2.9 percent, the contribution rate is 9.3 percent of earnings with population weighting and 8.9 percent with mortality weighting. When the higher discount rate of 5.2 percent is used, the two contribution rates fall to 4.0 percent and 3.8 percent with population and mortality weighting, respectively.

With this background, we now turn to the contribution-rate estimates that our data allow us to make for birth years 1933–2000. Given that the estimates are based on forecasted earnings and Medicare benefits as projected by the trustees, they are indicative of forecasted outcomes, not actual outcomes. Figure 10-3 depicts the contribution rates necessary to prepay Current Medicare benefits, net of premium payments, using mortality and population weighting, based on a 2.9 percent real rate of return. As expected, the rates based on the mortality weights are lower than those based on population weighting.[3]

Figure 10-4 makes the same comparison with the contribution rates based on a real return of 5.2 percent. Together, the two graphs provide a range of reasonable estimates of the cost of prepayment by birth year. It is evident from both that scheduled lifetime net Medicare benefits are growing relative to lifetime earnings for successive groups of new retirees. The rates may appear to be high relative to the current HI payroll tax rate of 2.9 percent, even with the higher discount rate, but recall that the calculated rates prepay all of Medicare—Parts A, B, and D—net of premiums for Parts B and D. As an additional point of reference, note that the long-run actuarial deficit for Part A alone is 5.8 percent of taxable payroll, and if the actuarial deficits of Parts B and D are cast as percentages of payroll, the total Medicare actuarial

---

3. In the two cases in which the contribution rates are almost identical, for birth years 1942 and 1947, the net effects of new entrants due to immigration and their associated mortality rates are smaller than for the later birth years.

FIGURE 10-3

CONTRIBUTION RATES SUFFICIENT TO PREPAY CURRENT MEDICARE AS
PERCENTAGES OF EARNINGS, BY BIRTH YEAR
Government Bond Rate of 2.9 Percent Assumed

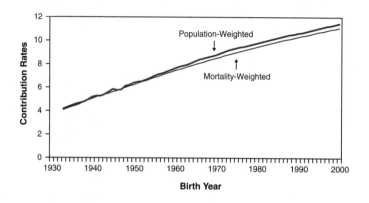

SOURCE: Authors' estimates.

FIGURE 10-4

CONTRIBUTION RATES SUFFICIENT TO PREPAY CURRENT MEDICARE AS
PERCENTAGES OF EARNINGS, BY BIRTH YEAR
60/40 Portfolio Rate of 5.2 Percent Assumed

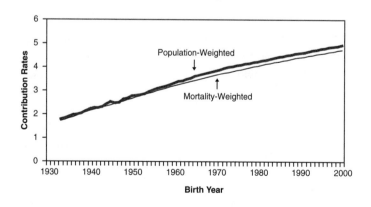

SOURCE: Authors' estimates.

deficit is 14.5 percent of taxable payroll. Adding in the 2.9 percent payroll tax produces a cost of 17.4 percent of taxable payroll. This is the tax rate required this year, and every subsequent year, to fund Medicare indefinitely using a single trust fund.[4]

The contribution rates depicted in figures 10-3 and 10-4 assume contributions beginning at the age of eighteen and continuing until seventy. The estimates are presented to illustrate the prepayment rates that would have been necessary to pay the benefits each cohort is expected to receive. For the younger cohorts—those born in 1988 and later—the rates are indicative of the cost of prepayment from 2006 and later for future labor-force entrants. As we turn our attention in the next chapter to a transition to prepaid Medicare, we will use the contribution rates calculated here as the basis for the funding requirements during this transition.

The estimated contribution rates can also be used to compare prepayment to the current pay-as-you-go financing arrangement and thus determine which generations are net beneficiaries of, or net contributors to, Medicare. Individuals in birth cohorts for whom the required prepayment contribution rate is greater than the lifetime Medicare taxes they pay, or will pay, are net beneficiaries of the system. Those in cohorts who face higher taxes than the required contributions are net payers into the system. The initial Part A beneficiaries who turned sixty-five when the program first started paying benefits were clearly net beneficiaries. They paid no payroll taxes but received benefits over their remaining lifetimes. The contribution rate we would calculate for them, as the ratio of the present value of benefits to earnings, would be positive and clearly in excess of their lifetime tax rate of zero.

Figure 10-5 compares lifetime tax rates to contribution rates. In order to calculate lifetime Medicare taxes we were required to make some simplifying assumptions. In each year we calculated a total net Medicare tax, which is equal to the ratio of total scheduled Medicare spending, net of Parts B and D premiums, to taxable payroll. While this tax rate ignores the fact that Parts B and D are paid through general revenues, it is the appropriate complement to the way in which we calculated the required contribution rates.[5] These annual tax rates are applied to the earnings profiles to arrive at the present value of taxes as a percentage of present-value earnings, which is an estimate

---

4. We discuss this estimate further in chapter 12.

FIGURE 10-5
LIFETIME CURRENT MEDICARE TAXES AND CONTRIBUTION RATES AS
PERCENTAGES OF EARNINGS, BY BIRTH YEAR
Polulation Weighting

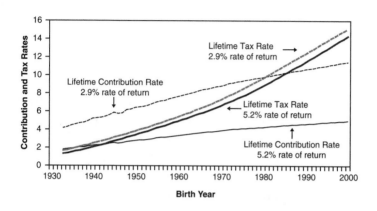

SOURCE: Authors' estimates.

of the lifetime Medicare tax rate. The tax rates and contribution rates, based on population weighting, are given in figure 10-5 using the two rates-of-return assumptions, 2.9 percent and 5.2 percent. The contribution-rate schedules are taken from figures 10-3 and 10-4.

The lower rate-of-return assumption of 2.9 percent produces the higher contribution- and tax-rate schedules in the figure. The lifetime tax rates range from 1.6 percent to 15.1 percent for individuals born in 1933 and 2000, respectively, while the contribution rates range from 4.1 percent to 11.4 percent. To put the lifetime tax rates in perspective, note that individuals born in 1933 did not start paying for Medicare until they reached the age of thirty-three in 1966. Their Medicare tax was thus zero between the ages of nineteen and thirty-two, and they also then paid very low taxes in the early years of the program. By the time individuals in the 1933 birth

---

5. This calculation of the tax rate for each year brings the tax burden associated with Parts B and D financing forward in a cohort's lifetime. However, income taxes that would have been paid during a cohort's retirement years are not included.

cohort were eligible in 1998, Medicare's net costs were 4.5 percent of payroll. Individuals born in 2000, however, will face annual tax rates ranging from 8.0 percent, when they are eighteen years of age, to, ultimately, 19.9 percent in the year prior to retirement. With the higher return, the tax rates range from 1.3 percent to 14.2 percent, and the contribution rates range from 1.8 percent to 4.9 percent.

The crossover of lifetime contribution rates and lifetime tax rates indicates the birth year for which a prepayment system would be preferred. In figure 10-5, using the lower rate of return, we see that only individuals born in 1980 or after have higher lifetime tax rates than contribution rates, and would have been better off with prepayment. As the assumed rate of return increases, the crossover moves backward in time. Thus, with the higher-return assumption, individuals born in 1942 and later would have been better off with prepayment.

Figure 10-6 presents the ratio of lifetime Medicare benefits to lifetime Medicare taxes by birth year. The ratio falls as birth year rises, independent of the rate of return assumed. Individuals in birth years for whom lifetime benefits are in excess of lifetime taxes have ratios above one, indicating they are net beneficiaries of the current method of Medicare financing. A ratio of less than one identifies cohorts that are net taxpayers into Medicare. As the figure shows, the rate of return matters.

All birth cohorts to the right of the unit-ratio crossover point are losers in the generational-transfer game. The most telling conclusion is that even with a rate of return at the low government borrowing rate, often considered the "risk-free net rate of return," those born in 1980 or later— anyone twenty-six or younger today—including all future taxpayers, will be net taxpayers into Medicare. Using the higher discount rate (justified if interpreted as the gross rate of return), the figure indicates that anyone born in 1942 or later—almost all current workers and all future taxpayers— will receive less in Medicare benefits than they pay in Medicare taxes. Thus, it is plausible to conclude that many members of the baby boom generation are net contributors to the program as well.[6]

---

6. See Auerbach, Kotlikoff, and Leibfritz (1999) for a discussion of the appropriate discount rate in generational accounting exercises like the one summarized in the figure. Also see Liu, Rettenmaier, and Saving (2005) for a discussion of the gross and net risk-free

FIGURE 10-6
RATIO OF LIFETIME CURRENT MEDICARE BENEFITS TO LIFETIME
CURRENT MEDICARE TAXES, BY BIRTH YEAR
Polulation Weighting

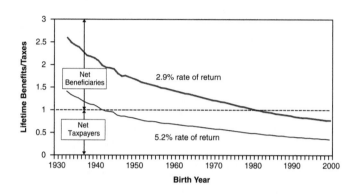

SOURCE: Authors' estimates.

## Conclusion

In this chapter we have estimated the contribution rate required to pre-pay Current Medicare, assuming the real rate of return assumed by the Medicare trustees and a rate of return more relevant for economy-wide real investment of the prepayment funds. One way to compare the contribution rates and lifetime tax rates is to review those required by the 2000 birth cohort, the most recent for which we can make estimates. In figure 10-7 we show, for the 2000 cohort, the contribution rate required to prepay Current Medicare and the lifetime tax rate that would be required to pay for a Current Medicare financed by generational transfer.

For both rates of return, the 2000 birth cohort is better off with pre-paid Medicare than Medicare financed by generational transfer. At the

---

rates of return and their applications. Earlier we identified the 5.2 percent rate of return as opportunity cost of funds for individuals. It can also be considered the "risk-free gross rate of return" if the corporate taxes are added to the government borrowing rate.

FIGURE 10-7

CONTRIBUTION RATES AND LIFETIME TAX RATES: PREPAID VERSUS
GENERATION-TRANSFER-FINANCED CURRENT MEDICARE,
2000 BIRTH COHORT BY RATE OF RETURN

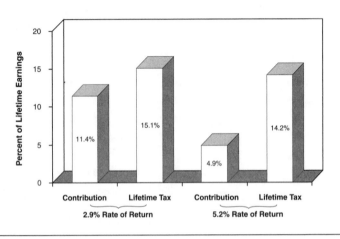

SOURCE: Authors' estimates.

more relevant real rate of return, 5.2 percent, the lifetime tax rate required
to pay for Current Medicare is almost three times the prepayment contribution rate. We should point out the obvious here, however. We know
that prepayment dominates generational-transfer financing for all
younger cohorts, even with very low assumed real rates of return. The
problem is that for older or perhaps even middle-aged cohorts, the transition will require sacrifices that will outweigh the difference between the
prepaid contribution rate and the lifetime tax rate.

Perhaps the issue, however, is not about Current Medicare, since it is
clearly unsustainable, but about a new Medicare that must eventually be
put in place. While we do not know what that Medicare will be, we can
evaluate the reforms that we scored in chapters 5–8. In the next chapter,
we estimate the contribution rates necessary to fund these reforms.

# 11

# Prepaying Reformed Medicare Benefits

To this point we have discussed prepaying Medicare benefits as they are currently forecast by the Medicare trustees. Since Current Medicare is not sustainable in the long run, we now consider the cost of prepaying the four reforms outlined in chapters 5–8. Naturally, the contribution rates necessary to fund the various reformed programs will be lower than those required to prepay benefits as currently predicted. But, as discussed earlier, these lower costs are only those that are accounted for as government spending. Beneficiaries will have additional costs, as they will be responsible for the difference between the trustees' projected total Medicare expenditures and the cost of the reformed programs, except in the case of No-First-Dollar Medicare, which is the only reform for which we specifically account for reduced health-care expenditures.

In addition, each of the reforms could affect the incentives of beneficiaries. Therefore, the total health-care spending of future retirees under each reform may differ from the trustees' projections, along with the lifetime costs of each option. The expected result of the scaled-back transfers retirees would receive with each reform is a reduction in health-care utilization by the elderly as they face higher cost-sharing. Such reductions are efficient if they eliminate the consumption of services whose marginal costs exceed their marginal benefits. In the present exercise we do not attempt to account for the degree to which the various reforms affect lifetime welfare for each cohort.

In the next chapter we are primarily concerned with illustrating how the reforms would affect the timing of the costs borne by taxpayers. In the case of prepayment, the costs include taxpayers' contributions to retirement health-insurance accounts and the costs of paying Medicare benefits to current retirees and part of the costs for future retirees who have not fully prepaid their retirement health care. The cohort-specific contribution rates identified in this chapter will be used in the next chapter to account for these additional upfront costs of prepayment.

Figure 11-1 shows the contribution rates associated with the reforms scored in chapters 5 and 6—Commission Medicare, 2011 Technology Medicare, and Retirement Technology Medicare. For comparative purposes, we also show in figure 11-1 the contribution rates necessary to prepay currently projected benefits. For simplicity, we use mortality-weighted estimates to illustrate the relative contribution rates, and we assume that the real rate of return is the government borrowing rate of 2.9 percent.[1] Raising the retirement age to sixty-seven produces the smallest reduction in contribution rates. As can be seen in the figure, we implemented this reform in two discrete steps rather than applying the actual, more gradual, increase in the normal retirement age scheduled for Social Security.[2] From the lifetime spending profiles, we know that spending at sixty-five and sixty-six is relatively low; consequently, the reductions in the contribution rates associated with this reform are modest.

The relative shapes of the contribution-rate profiles for the two fixed-technology reforms result from our specific implementation of the reforms. Both begin in 2011, when the oldest members of the baby boom generation—individuals born in 1946—reach sixty-five, the age of Medicare eligibility. In both cases, actual spending between 2006 and 2011 by individuals born prior to 1946 is identical to projected spending, but is then capped at the real age-spending profile in 2011.

---

1. Recall that population weighting produces slightly higher estimates for each birth cohort. We use mortality weighting to define the contribution rates. The rates are calculated assuming participation in prepayment from the year the cohort enters the labor force. We implicitly assume that workers who enter the labor force later in life or who enter as immigrants must make up for past contributions to be eligible for full benefits at retirement. In our estimates in the next chapter of the transition to prepayment, we use the population-weighted contribution rates to define the total costs of the transition.

2. The current "normal" retirement age for Social Security is sixty-six and is scheduled to begin rising by one month per year in 2010, until reaching sixty-seven years of age in 2022.

FIGURE 11-1
PREPAYMENT CONTRIBUTION RATES: CURRENT, COMMISSION,
RETIREMENT TECHNOLOGY, AND 2011 TECHNOLOGY
MEDICARE PERCENTAGES OF EARNINGS, BY BIRTH YEAR
Mortality-Weighted and a 2.9 Percent Rate of Return Assumed

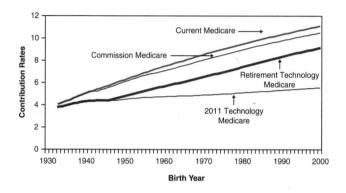

SOURCE: Authors' estimates.

With the reform that fixes Medicare transfers to the technology that exists in the year an individual reaches retirement age, the contribution rates rise less rapidly than those associated with prepaying Current Medicare projected benefits. The contribution rate grows from 4.35 percent of earnings for individuals born in 1946 to 9.07 percent for individuals born in 2000.[3] Recall that this option provides real benefits equal to the spending profile that exists in a birth cohort's retirement year.

The more aggressive form of the fixed-technology reform fixes the transfers to beneficiaries as defined by the age-spending profile that is currently projected for the year 2011. This profile is then indexed by real per-capita GDP growth to the year of retirement for cohorts retiring after 2011. Once a cohort's beginning age-spending profile is determined, it is subsequently price-level-adjusted using only the Consumer Price Index

---

3. Using the higher 5.2 percent real rate of return reflecting workers' opportunity cost of capital produces contribution rates of 2.88 percent and 5.99 percent, for the 1946 and 2000 birth cohorts, respectively.

(CPI)—that is, it is adjusted for general inflation, not health-care cost inflation. As implemented, this reform requires the same 4.35 percent contribution rate as Retirement Technology Medicare for individuals born in 1946 but a lower rate for all later cohorts, rising to 5.56 percent for individuals born in 2000.

Figure 11-2 shows the contribution rates associated with the two reforms outlined in chapters 7 and 8, No-First-Dollar Medicare and Means-Tested Medicare. The contribution rates necessary to prepay Current Medicare projected benefits are again presented for comparison. Both of these reforms produce contribution-rate profiles roughly proportional to scheduled benefits. Means-Tested Medicare results in contribution rates about 80 percent of the size of those necessary to prepay Current Medicare scheduled benefits. The high-deductible policy, No-First-Dollar Medicare, results in contribution rates 63 percent of the size of those required to fund scheduled benefits.

Once again, we have to bear in mind that these two reforms in particular have significant incentive effects. For No-First-Dollar Medicare, we

FIGURE 11-2

PREPAYMENT CONTRIBUTION RATES: CURRENT, NO-FIRST-DOLLAR, AND
MEANS-TESTED MEDICARE PERCENTAGES OF EARNINGS, BY BIRTH YEAR

Mortality-Weighted and a 2.9 Percent Rate of Return Assumed

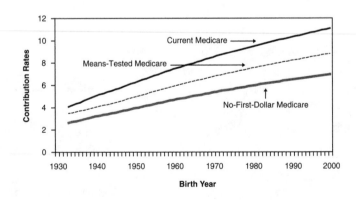

SOURCE: Authors' estimates.

explicitly take these incentive effects into account. However, for Means-Tested Medicare, the estimates assume that the high-income, and therefore low-benefit, beneficiaries, will not opt out of the system. Should they opt out, their marginal costs of care will likely rise, and we can expect that their health-care expenditures will be lower than those projected by the trustees.

## Additional Concerns

Since we first proposed prepaying Medicare in 1998 (see Gramm, Rettenmaier, and Saving [1998]), several concerns have been raised related to the particular form of prepayment we outlined. We previously proposed that prepaying retirement health care be done on a cohort-by-cohort basis with individualized insurance contracts, that participation be mandatory, and that cohort members buy health insurance in the private market at retirement.

The costs of the transition to prepayment from the current generational-transfer regime, as outlined in the next chapter, are primarily borne by the current working generation, which is expected to begin funding retirement health savings accounts at the cohort-specific rates reflected in figures 11-1 and 11-2. In addition, these workers must pay for the Medicare spending of current retirees. Further, for the entirety of the transition phase—that is, until all retirees' health-care spending is fully prepaid—some tax revenues will be necessary.[4] The tax requirement will decline as more and more retirees in future years have built up funds in their retirement health-insurance accounts.

The benefits of prepayment, in the form of lower taxes, higher savings and income, and a reduction in the common-pool problems associated with the current open-ended, in-kind transfer, accrue to future generations. Though the benefits arguably outweigh the costs, convincing the current gen-

---

4. As mentioned, the contribution rates identified in figures 11-1 and 11-2 are calculated using the conservative government borrowing rate. A higher return assumption is justified if all taxes, including corporate, are waived on the account accumulations. Also, for the older cohorts in 2006, contributions at the rates suggested in this chapter will prepay a small fraction of retirement health care. Only the new entrants to the labor force in 2006 and the cohorts that follow will fully prepay their retirement health-care consumption.

eration to bear a higher funding burden has been the bane of anyone pro-posing prepayment of current transfers to the elderly. In the next chapter, in which we discuss the transition to prepayment, all costs are accounted for in the year they are incurred. That is, the taxes necessary to pay non-prepaid benefits to current and future retirees, as well as the costs of funding retire-ment health-insurance accounts, are recognized each year. In this way, the change in the annual total cost rates and the generational consequences are clearly identified. Some of the transition cost could be distributed to future generations by borrowing, but given that the reforms we outline include reductions in the transfers relative to those that are currently projected, future generations of retirees are already sharing in this cost.

More specific concerns include the problem of within-generation vari-ation in earnings, which produces disparate account sizes at retirement. Further, differing health-care risks at retirement may produce the problems associated with adverse selection or screening on the part of insurers. Both are distributional concerns that are also present in the current financing arrangement.

Persuading voters to prepay—that is, to consume less now so that future workers will have a smaller implicit debt burden—is a public-choice issue. Current voters must decide which is more secure: a prepaid retirement insur-ance contract, or the hope that when they are old their Medicare benefits will not be reduced. A prepaid contract provides some assurance against the loss of health coverage, but as we know from the demographic projections, retirees will become a larger share of eligible voters in all years after the baby boom generation enters retirement. Prepaying Medicare is not the only pub-lic policy that benefits the next generation at the expense of current workers. The same logic of "current-generation sacrifice for future generations' well-being" is used in discussions of reducing explicit federal debts, preserving the environment, conserving fossil fuels, and reducing other implicit debts such as those associated with scheduled Social Security.

As to the distributional issues, we have purposefully outlined a general mechanism by which retirement health care is prepaid. Conceiving of the prepayment vehicle as a retirement health-insurance pension abstracts from some of the distributional concerns associated with individual retirement health accounts. In this way, any concerns about within-generation varia-tion in earnings and in benefit payouts during retirement are shared with

Current Medicare Part A. However, with prepayment, the contributions to the health-insurance pensions are invested in real resources rather than being distributed as benefits in the year they are received.

Further, the health-insurance pension providers would have to be independent from the federal government. At retirement, pension providers would pay a premium on behalf of each beneficiary to a private health insurer, or the health-insurance pension provider could also serve as a payer. Outside payments could be risk-adjusted, or, alternatively, assignment to other providers could be random, to overcome any selection issues.

Explicitly prepaying the five reformed programs may lead to questions concerning how health-care spending over and above the amount covered by the specific reforms is handled. The reforms to the benefit package will affect beneficiaries' budget constraints, and, ultimately, the time-path of total health-care consumption by the elderly, in different ways. We do not attempt to identify these incentive effects in our estimates, though all would tend to reduce total health-care spending relative to that forecast with the current institution. Spending in addition to the amounts covered by the reformed insurance would have to come from beneficiaries or contemporaneous transfers, or simply from reduced spending.

The means-testing reform is the most straightforward in how the funding would be handled. The transfers to lower-income retirees would remain the same, while higher-income retirees would have to spend from their own incomes. Apart from any formal prepayment, the reform by itself would induce individuals who anticipate high retirement income to respond by saving more, and thus implicitly prepay some of their retirement health-care consumption. Additionally, unless participation in the formally prepaid portion of the retirement health insurance is mandatory, workers with higher lifetime earnings would prefer to opt out rather than subsidize the other workers in their birth cohort. The other reforms will also elicit additional savings, assuming future retirees desire to spend more than the reformed transfer. Variation in retirement income and/or the degree to which workers respond to the reform with additional saving will potentially produce greater variation in health-care spending among retirees than currently exists.

Medicare's uniform insurance coverage across beneficiaries has, since its inception, been seen by many as one of its most important features. Those who defend uniform coverage suggest that moving away from it will reduce the widespread support of the program. This reasoning is often used in the rhetoric favoring universal health-care coverage across all age groups. We cannot resolve these equity concerns here, but the equity argument cuts both ways, both within and between generations.

Medicare awards uniform benefits to all eligible individuals. Some 97 percent of the elderly are covered by the program, so it is essentially universal health-care coverage for the aged. However, there is much variation among current retirees in the lifetime HI payroll taxes they paid and in the lifetime income taxes that they paid when working, or will pay during their retirement, to support Parts B and D spending. Thus, Current Medicare is actually quite unequal in its treatment of retirees within and across generations.

In the Social Security system, variation in lifetime earnings is overcome, in a limited way, by the redistribution inherent in the benefit formula that replaces a higher percentage of income for low lifetime earners than for high-income workers. Bear in mind, however, that the redistribution is limited to those who work the full number of years. Any worker who is in the labor force for very few years receives low benefits. As we have shown above with Medicare, some birth cohorts are net beneficiaries, and some are net payers into the program; consequently, Medicare is not "fair" across generations. In the long run, prepayment will bring about greater generational equity.

## Conclusion

In this chapter we have estimated the contribution rate required to prepay Current Medicare and the five reforms we scored in chapters 5–8. One way to compare the contribution rates is to review that required by the 2000 birth cohort, the most recent for which we could make an estimate. In figure 11-3 we see that the contribution rates for the 2000 birth cohort range from 11.0 percent for Current Medicare to 5.6 percent for 2011 Technology Medicare.[5] In making this comparison it is important to bear in mind that these contributions do not represent the full cost of retirement

---

5. Using the higher 5.2 percent real rate of return produces a range of contribution rates between 7.2 percent and 3.7 percent for Current Medicare and 2011 Technology Medicare, respectively.

health care. Each reformed Medicare, with the exception of No-First-Dollar Medicare, requires that retirees also prepay the difference between the level of health care provided by the particular reform in question and their own desired level of health care. The estimate for Current Medicare provides an upper bound of the required prepayment contribution rates.

FIGURE 11-3
BIRTH-YEAR 2000 CONTRIBUTION RATES: ALL REFORMS
2.9 Percent Rate of Return Assumed

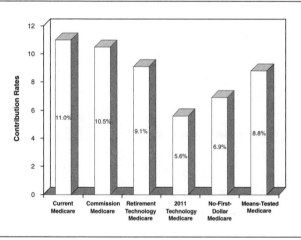

SOURCE: Authors' estimates.

While the transition to a generational-transfer system of financing retirement health care was easy in 1965, undoing the system is difficult. The difficulty arises because, in the initial transition to the generational-transfer system, no living member of society was worse off; only unborn members suffered. They suffered because the transfer-payment system reduces the need to save for retirement consumption, and, as a result, the capital stock is lower than it would be in the absence of generational-transfer payments. The transition back, however, will affect currently living members of society. What we have done in this chapter is to price prepaid Medicare for both the existing program and the reformed programs outlined in chapters 5–8. We leave the discussion of how the transition can be accomplished to the next chapter.

# 12

# The Transition to Prepaid
# Retirement Health Insurance

Moving from transfer-payment financing to prepaid financing of Medicare requires that current workers begin prepaying their future health care while at the same time paying the necessary taxes in support of the transfers to current beneficiaries. A convenient way to introduce the concept of prepayment can be found in the *2006 Medicare Trustees Report*. Each year, the dollar value of the HI funding shortfall, along with the shortfall expressed as a percentage of taxable earnings, is presented for two time horizons: the next seventy-five years and the indefinite future. When the shortfall is expressed as a percentage of taxable earnings, the ratio is referred to as the actuarial balance.

According to the trustees' definition,

> The actuarial balance can be interpreted as the percentage points that must be added to the current law income rates and/or subtracted from the current law cost rates immediately and throughout the entire valuation period in order for the financing to support HI costs and provide for the targeted trust fund balance at the end of the projection period.[1]

Thus, adding the respective actuarial balances to the current income rates results in the tax rates that will support HI for seventy-five years or for the indefinite future.

---

1. The *2006 Annual Report of the Boards of Trustees of the Federal Hospital Insurance and Federal Supplementary Medical Insurance Trust Funds*, 59.

For the actuarial balance to be meaningful, any excess revenues or surpluses generated when current tax rates are above the current cost rate must provide the resources for future spending. If current surpluses are to be available in the future, they must be saved in the form of claims on real resources; they cannot be spent on other federal projects. If the surpluses are stored as savings, this would represent a form of partial prepayment through the trust fund.

Based on the 2006 report, the seventy-five-year HI actuarial deficit is three and a half percentage points. The current HI income rate as a percentage of payroll is 3.39 percent, which is the sum of the 2.9 percent HI payroll tax rate and the revenue from the taxation of Social Security benefits. This income rate, plus the actuarial deficit of three and a half percentage points, would be necessary to make the system solvent for the next seventy-five years. When the actuarial deficit is combined with a summary measure of the current seventy-five-year income rate of 3.39 percent of taxable payroll, the total tax bill sufficient to fund the HI portion of Medicare is 6.90 percent. To fund HI over the indefinite horizon would require additional tax revenues equal to 5.8 percent of taxable payroll, resulting in an 8.70 percent tax rate on payroll.

But either of these much higher payroll tax rates would only pay for the HI portion of Medicare. The rates required to fund all parts of Medicare over the next seventy-five years and the indefinite horizon are given in table 12-1. Adding in the funding requirements of Medicare's Supplementary Medical Insurance (SMI; Parts B and D) ups the payroll tax to 13.0 percent to fund all of Medicare over the next seventy-five years through the trust fund and to 17.5 percent to pay for the program indefinitely. By way of comparison, the payroll tax rate required to fund all of Medicare on a continual-flow basis was given in chapter 3. There we indicated that at the close of the trustees' seventy-five-year projection period, the payroll tax rate would have to be 19.2 percent, significantly higher than the 13.0 percent cited above. The difference is that the 13.0 percent tax rate must begin now and continue for the next seventy-five years, whereas the contemporaneous tax rate would only reach the 13.0 percent level in 2043 and then continue rising for all the years thereafter.

Denominating the actuarial balances for all parts of Medicare by taxable payroll should not be interpreted as suggesting a policy to implement this. It

TABLE 12-1
PAYROLL TAX RATES NECESSARY TO FUND MEDICARE
BENEFITS THROUGH TRUST FUNDS

|  | Hospital Insurance | Net of SMI Premiums Supplementary Medical Insurance | | |
|---|---|---|---|---|
|  | Part A | Part B | Part D | Total |
| 75-year | 6.4 | 4.1 | 2.5 | 13.0 |
| Indefinite Horizon | 8.7 | 5.4 | 3.3 | 17.4 |

SOURCES: Authors' estimates and *2006 Medicare Trustees Report*, Table III.B11.

is used here as a way to denominate all of the deficits in a common way. Paying for all Medicare spending via a payroll tax affects both the within- and between-generational burdens. The SMI funding requirements could also be denominated as a percentage of historical nonentitlement revenues, as we did in chapter 3. Our ultimate purpose here is to illustrate the mechanics of prepayment on a cohort-by-cohort basis, and denominating all Medicare spending relative to taxable payroll allows for a comparison to the current arrangement. Ideally, a move to prepayment would be coupled with a more efficient tax regime, such as a consumption tax. In this way the accrued retirement health-care benefits of current retirees and of current workers who cannot fully prepay their benefits would be paid for through a tax that imposes the burden across age groups until the non-prepaid benefits are retired.

## A Point of Reference: Achieving Actuarial Balance through Trust-Fund Financing

The object of the current exercise is to point out the implications of partially prepaying Medicare through a single trust fund. All workers would pay a 17.5 percent tax rate that would remain constant for all future years and suffice to pay benefits to both the disabled and aged Medicare beneficiaries indefinitely. Given that we are only interested in prepaying retirement health-care consumption, the necessary tax rate is less.[2] We estimate that a permanent payroll tax rate of 15.4 percent would suffice to pay Medicare benefits for the retired population indefinitely, provided the additional tax revenues are equal to the 12.5 percent of payroll required to pay aged Medicare benefits indefinitely. The constant 15.4 percent rate combined with the HI revenues from taxation of benefits is depicted in figure 12-1, alongside Medicare's total annual costs in support of aged beneficiaries, net of SMI premiums.[3]

The costs depicted in the figure are those that must be paid from tax revenues, whatever the sources of those revenues. To eliminate the actuarial deficit, revenues must average 15.4 percent of HI taxable payroll annually. As

FIGURE 12-1
CURRENT MEDICARE INCOME AND COST-RATES BENEFICIARIES,
AGES SIXTY-FIVE AND OLDER
Income Rate Necessary to Pay Costs Indefinitely through a Single Trust Fund

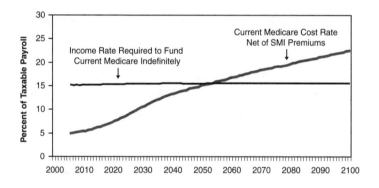

SOURCE: Authors' estimates.
NOTE: Cost rate is total Medicare spending on the aged net of premium payments as a percent of HI taxable payroll. Income rate is current-law HI income apportioned to the aged and the combined HI and SMI actuarial deficit.

2. In a real sense, the transfers to the disabled are within-generation transfers and not between-generation transfers. The benefits of prepayment accrue only to the elimination of between-generation transfers.

3. HI payroll taxes are divided between the disabled and the aged based on the two groups' respective proportions of total spending in each year.

the income and cost rates indicate, the system would experience surpluses until 2053. Thereafter, the deficits would be covered by the trust fund, which would never be exhausted. Initially, the surplus would amount to 10.2 percent of taxable payroll, or double the size of current net Medicare spending on the aged. Because the permanent tax rate is above that which would be required for full prepayment, even in the steady state (recall from the previous chapter that the contribution rate of the 2000 birth cohort was estimated to be 11 percent), this system has a component of between-generation transfer-payment financing. Because the rate is immediately increased, the tax burden is shifted forward to older workers in that they would pay a higher tax rate than currently scheduled and therefore pay for some part of the transition.

Achieving actuarial balance by raising the payroll tax rate immediately by 12.5 percent means that all new entrants to the labor force pay the new higher, constant tax rate throughout their lives. The lifetime tax burden on current workers would fall as we move up the age distribution, given that the higher rate imposed beginning in 2006 would affect older workers only toward the ends of their careers, and these workers would have only slightly higher lifetime tax rates than those based on a continuation of the current transfer-payment financing.

In sum, to prepay through a single trust fund requires initial income in excess of expenditures so as to build up reserves. Partial prepayment of this type also shifts the tax burden forward to current older workers. However, as the contribution rates estimated in the previous chapter illustrated, the cohort-by-cohort lifetime tax rates under the current program do not coincide with the lifetime contribution rates necessary to prepay Medicare. Younger cohorts would have to contribute more because their Medicare consumption will be larger than that of older cohorts and will represent a larger share of their preretirement earnings.

## A Transition Path to Prepaid Medicare

Because health-care consumption is growing faster than lifetime earnings, the prepayment of retirement health care will require higher contribution rates as time goes on. Ideally, all cohorts would receive benefits equal to the accumulated value of their contributions, and the system would be neutral in its treatment of generations. Moving to a prepaid system would begin with each new group of labor market entrants contributing to a retirement health-care pension at an actuarially fair rate. The contributions would be at the mortality-weighted rates discussed in the previous chapter. Individuals who enter the prepaid plans at later ages would have to make up for past payments. Our estimates implicitly assume that members of any given birth cohort pay the same contribution rate, producing within-generation redistribution from higher-paid members of the cohort to lower-paid members each year, and throughout the cohort's years in the labor force.

We analyze the prepayment path for all of the reforms previously outlined, evaluating them as follows: Workers ages eighteen and over would contribute to a retirement health-insurance pension at the rate that would have fully prepaid, net of premium, their retirement benefits had their cohort contributed beginning at age eighteen.[4] This contribution rate would prepay only a small portion of the retirement health-care consumption of older current workers, but would fully repay it for current eighteen-year-old workers, who were born in 1988, net of premiums.[5] Thus, with this transition framework, all birth cohorts born in 1988 and later would fully prepay their retirement health insurance. In addition to the contributions to their prepaid retirement health insurance, all workers would pay the remaining costs of the current system for current retirees and for the retirement health-care costs of current workers that are not prepaid through the cohort-specific contribution rates.

This transition framework is similar to one often used to evaluate transitions to fully or partially prepaid Social Security—namely, contribution rates to personal retirement accounts are often identical across workers, with older workers, at the outset of the reform, accumulating less

---

4. Importantly, each cohort's contribution rate in this transition framework is the actuarially fair contribution rate, assuming lifetime contributions, that would have funded its retirement health-care net of premium payments had the cohort begun contributing when it entered the labor force.

5. Workers do not prepay total spending but, rather, spending less premiums. For the status quo, the premiums are exactly as projected, approximately 25 percent of Part B and 23 percent of Part D spending. For the other reforms these percentages continue to hold, but the total spending is less, and thus the dollar amounts of premiums are less than status quo spending.

in their accounts by the time they retire than younger workers. The older workers have fewer years to contribute to their retirement accounts and would thus prepay less of their scheduled Social Security benefits. Similarly, at the outset of the reform, the older workers in our examples would be able to prepay less of their retirement health care than the younger workers. And, as noted, an increasing contribution rate for the younger and younger cohorts is appropriate in the case of prepaying Medicare, given the increasing size of the transfer for successive groups of retirees.

As we have seen from the example of partial prepayment through a single trust fund, prepayment requires higher initial annual revenue flows and eliminates the system's unfunded obligation and actuarial deficit. Full prepayment on a cohort-by-cohort basis also eliminates the unfunded obligation, but, as we will see, the timing of the costs is different; and, ultimately, the long-run cost rates are lower.

The effects of full prepayment can be summarized graphically by the cost and revenue flows and by measures of the unfunded obligations. Our examples present the annual flows, and from them the unfunded obligations are calculated, along with several other summary measures. A set of figures based on prepaying Current Medicare provides some context for the summary measures presented later for each of the reforms and under various rate-of-return assumptions.

We begin by considering examples of the system's long-run cost and revenue flows before prepayment. Next, we depict examples of the cost and revenue flows associated with the closed group, or those individuals who are current beneficiaries and/or current taxpayers. These costs and revenues are relevant for the discussion of our implementation of prepayment, given that all new entrants to the program after 2006 will fully prepay their net retirement health-care consumption.

Figure 12-2 shows the annual costs and revenues for Current Medicare and for Retirement Technology Medicare. The costs are limited to beneficiaries ages sixty-five and over, and the revenues are again those apportioned to the aged. This graph shows that, as a result of the reform, costs are reduced to a greater extent than revenues. The only difference between Current Medicare and Retirement Technology Medicare revenues is the reduction in the premiums resulting from the reduced-benefit awards. Benefit taxes and payroll taxes remain the same. The seventy-five-year open-group unfunded liability is $27.8 trillion for Current Medicare and $20.6 trillion for Retirement Technology Medicare. These shortfalls are referred to as the seventy-five-year open-group unfunded obligation because the group is open to new participants, initially as taxpayers and ultimately as beneficiaries.

FIGURE 12-2

OPEN-GROUP EXPENDITURES AND INCOME:
CURRENT AND RETIREMENT TECHNOLOGY MEDICARE
Beneficiaries 65 and Older

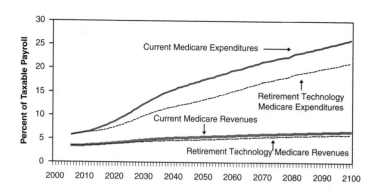

SOURCE: Authors' estimates. Revenues include HI payroll taxes, benefit taxes, and premium payments apportioned to aged beneficiaries.

The closed-group unfunded obligations are derived from the Current Medicare and Retirement Technology Medicare flows shown in figure 12-3 (on the following page). The costs and revenues are limited to those associated with members of the closed group, individuals eighteen and older in 2006. Relative to the revenues depicted in figure 12-2, the revenues shown here do not include the payroll taxes paid by individuals born after 1988. In later years, when individuals born in 1989 and after retire, the revenues do not include their benefit taxes or their premium payments.

Ultimately, closed-group revenues decline to zero, along with their costs. The fact that the group is closed to new entrants is seen by the two

FIGURE 12-3
CLOSED-GROUP EXPENDITURES AND INCOME:
CURRENT AND RETIREMENT TECHNOLOGY MEDICARE
Beneficiaries 65 and Older

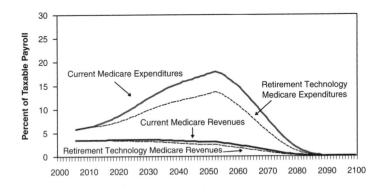

SOURCE: Authors' estimates. Revenues include HI payroll taxes, benefit taxes, and premium payments apportioned to aged beneficiaries who are members of the closed group .

cost-paths. Between 2006 and 2053, the closed-group cost rates are identical to the open-group rates because only retirees draw benefits, and, until 2053, all beneficiaries are members of the closed group. But in 2054, individuals born in 1989, who are not members of the closed group, retire. In that year, the closed-group and open-group costs diverge. With attrition, the closed-group costs decline to zero by the time today's eighteen-year-olds reach one hundred years of age, in 2088.[6] The closed-group unfunded obligation for aged beneficiaries is $25.8 trillion for Current Medicare and $19.5 trillion—24 percent less—for Retirement Technology Medicare.

Given that the transition path we analyze involves full prepayment of all cohorts born in 1988 and later and partial prepayment for today's

---

6. Technically, the hundred-year closed-group costs should extend beyond when the youngest cohort reaches one hundred years of age. The 2006 Social Security Administration population counts we use end at that age. Rather than distributing the survivors at age one hundred to later ages using the Social Security life tables, we limit the closed-group calculation to 2088.

FIGURE 12-4

**CURRENT MEDICARE COST RATES NET OF BENEFICIARY PREMIUMS**
Beneficiaries 65 and Older

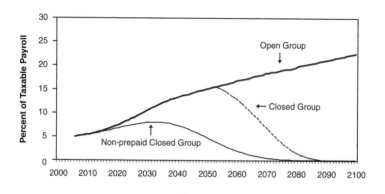

SOURCE: Authors' estimates. Non-prepaid Closed Group calculated assuming prepaid retirement insurance earns a rate of return equal to the government borrowing rate.

older workers, the annual taxpayer costs are limited to those associated with the closed group. These costs are depicted in figure 12-4 and, for illustrative purposes, shown only for Current Medicare.

The open-group and closed-group net-of-premium costs shown in the figure are derived from components in figures 12-2 and 12-3. Net-of-premium costs are those that must be paid annually by taxpayers. They are the difference between the annual expenditures in the previous graphs and the annual premiums that are included as components of annual revenues. The present value of Current Medicare's net-of-premium costs over the next seventy-five years is $36.9 trillion, and Current Medicare's closed-group cost is $30.4 trillion. The difference between these costs and the unfunded obligations are the respective payroll taxes paid by each group. The closed-group costs can be thought of as the accrued benefits owed to current participants, net of the premiums they are paying or will pay in their retirement. That is, if Current Medicare were closed today to new entrants born after 1988, the system would have a debt equal to $30.4 trillion, payable to current participants.

These accrued benefits are exactly the Current Medicare benefits that must be paid off during the transition to full prepayment. The final line in the figure shows the non-prepaid closed-group costs if prepayment begins in 2006. To allow for direct comparison with Current Medicare costs and the tax rate that achieves actuarial balance, these costs are calculated assuming the government borrowing rate of return of 2.9 percent, and are what remain of the closed-group cost as prepaid retirement health insurance replaces Current Medicare. Because each cohort in the closed group has a different number of years of remaining work life, individuals will prepay different percentages of their net Medicare benefits. Altogether, prepayment will result in non-prepaid costs that reach a maximum of 7.93 percent of payroll in 2032.

Workers begin contributing to prepaid retirement health-insurance plans at a rate that would have fully prepaid their retirement health insurance had they contributed at that rate from age eighteen. In table 12-2, we report the degree to which these contribution rates prepay net Medicare benefits for various ages of workers in the closed group. Younger workers prepay more of their retirement health-insurance consumption than older workers and have higher contribution rates, as seen in table 12-2.

Younger workers have higher lifetime contribution rates, since we have fixed the rate for each cohort in the closed group at that which, if paid from age eighteen to retirement at age sixty-five, would have funded their retirement health-care consumption.[7] Further, the greater number of years in the labor force for the younger cohorts in the closed group accounts for their higher percentage of full prepayment. In this example, and with the low government borrowing rate, the contribution rates range from 5.97 percent for individuals who are fifty-five years of age in 2006 to 10.43 percent for today's eighteen-year-old workers. The new entrants prepay 100 percent of net Medicare benefits, while the fifty-five-year-old individuals can pay for 16.9 percent of their benefits.

---

7. The contribution rates in table 12-2 are calculated using population rather than mortality weights for the prepayment simulations. While lifetime members of each cohort would contribute at the slightly lower mortality-weighted contribution rates, the population-weighted rates include the costs of new entrants to the system through immigration and are the relevant costs to compare to pay-as-you-go costs.

TABLE 12-2
CONTRIBUTION RATES AND PERCENTAGES OF NET MEDICARE
BENEFITS PREPAID BETWEEN 2006 AND RETIREMENT

| Age in 2006 | Contribution Rate | Percentage of Net Medicare Benefits Prepaid |
|---|---|---|
| 18 | 10.43 | 100.00 |
| 25 | 9.80 | 92.75 |
| 35 | 8.87 | 68.63 |
| 45 | 7.71 | 41.39 |
| 55 | 5.97 | 16.90 |

SOURCE: Authors' estimates.
NOTE: Contribution rate is determined using a 2.9 percent real rate of return.

Figure 12-5 (on the following page) allows us to compare three alternatives for paying net Medicare benefits. Each is designed to pay fully net Medicare benefits each year. Since most of the benefits accrue to future generations, they could participate in bearing some of the costs of prepayment by increased borrowing during the transition. However, such an option would postpone the benefits of prepayment—namely an increase in the capital stock—and, in the extreme, borrowing could leave the generational burden unchanged. Further, if any of the benefit-reducing reform options is adopted, these future generations will share the burden by receiving smaller lifetime benefits than those currently projected. The cost-rate series for the prepaid program is directly comparable to the income-rate series required to fund Medicare indefinitely through a single trust fund because both are calculated using the real 2.9 percent government borrowing rate. The graph clearly shows the relative tradeoffs of each approach.

The fully prepaid cost rate is arrived at by adding the non-prepaid closed-group costs, as shown in figure 12-4, to the population-weighted average of the different cohorts' contribution rates. Paying the cost rate on a contemporaneous basis defers the cost to the future. Achieving actuarial balance through partial prepayment with trust-fund financing produces relatively constant costs, with each generation of workers paying the same rate regardless of the relative size of their benefits. Like the trust fund route, full prepayment on a cohort-by-cohort basis has initially higher costs than pure pay-as-you-go financing, but, ultimately, the costs are lower and exactly equal to the benefits received.

FIGURE 12-5

ALTERNATIVE CURRENT MEDICARE COST RATES NET OF BENEFICIARY PREMIUMS, WITH AND WITHOUT PREPAYMENT
Beneficiaries 65 and Older

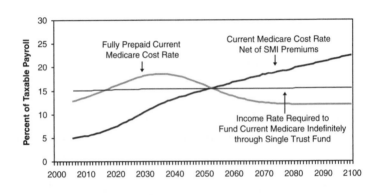

SOURCE: Authors' estimates. Prepaid cost rate and income rate required to fund Current Medicare indefinitely are both calculated assuming a rate of return equal to the government borrowing rate.

## Comparing Reforms under Alternative Rates of Return

Thus far we have only considered prepaying Current Medicare's net benefits assuming that the prepaid retirement health-insurance policies earn the government borrowing rate. However, rising health-care costs are likely to result in changes to Medicare's benefit structure along the lines of the reforms we have discussed. The preceding analysis provides points of reference for the comparison of reforms in this section, which assumes that the prepaid retirement health-insurance policies earn two alternative real rates of return: the government borrowing rate of 2.9 percent and the 60/40 stock/bond portfolio return of 5.2 percent. Tables 12-3 and 12-4 (on pages 138 and 139) summarize the reforms based on these respective rates. The estimates for Current Medicare are given in each table for comparison with the five reforms.

The top panel in each table reports summary present-value measures. All are calculated using the government borrowing rate and, as a result, the first four rows in each table are the same. Using table 12-3 as an example, the first two rows give the seventy-five-year open-group and hundred-year closed-group unfunded obligations, as reported in the previous two chapters. The annual flows underlying the present values were presented in figures 12-2 and 12-3 for Current Medicare and Retirement Technology Medicare. The third row reports the seventy-five-year open-group outgo, net of premiums. This is the present value of tax revenues necessary to fund the reform over the next seventy-five years. Each of the reforms has its expected effects on the seventy-five-year costs, with No-First-Dollar Medicare producing the greatest reduction. The next row gives the closed-group accrued benefits. Again, No-First-Dollar Medicare has the greatest effect in lowering the costs owed by taxpayers to current program participants. The annual net-of-premium costs associated with the open and closed group were illustrated in figure 12-4 for the status quo.

The values in the remainder of the tables are contingent on the rate of return applied to the prepaid retirement health-insurance policies. The next three rows summarize the effects of prepayment on the reforms' closed-group accrued benefits. The present values are again calculated using the government borrowing rate, but the rate of return earned on the prepaid retirement health-insurance policies combined with the contribution rates affect the amount of the closed group's accrued benefits that can be prepaid. Higher rates of return result in lower required lifetime contribution rates, and the combination results in lower shares of prepaid closed-group accrued benefits. This is evident when comparing the closed group's prepaid percentage of accrued benefits for Current Medicare across the two tables. The percentage of the closed group's accrued benefits that can be prepaid is 39.5 percent with the 5.2 percent return, from table 12-4, but is 45.3 percent with the lower 2.9 percent return, from table 12-3.

The last five rows of the tables summarize annual cost measures for each reform based on several critical values, as were illustrated in figure 12-5. The maximum prepayment cost rate and the year in which it is attained are given in the first two rows in the tables' lower panels. The maximum prepayment

TABLE 12-3

REFORM SUMMARY MEASURES—2.9 PERCENT REAL RATE OF RETURN

| Summary Measure | Present Value Measures (in billions) | | | | | |
|---|---|---|---|---|---|---|
| | Current | Commission | Retire Tech | 2011 Tech | Means-Test | No-First-Dollar |
| Open group unfunded | 27,769 | 26,119 | 20,645 | 14,787 | 20,089 | 14,034 |
| Closed group unfunded | 25,816 | 24,775 | 19,492 | 15,738 | 19,617 | 14,555 |
| Net open group outgo | 36,856 | 35,206 | 29,732 | 23,874 | 29,176 | 23,121 |
| Closed group accrued benefits | 30,387 | 29,346 | 24,064 | 20,309 | 24,188 | 19,126 |
| Non-prepaid closed group accrued benefits | 16,626 | 16,226 | 13,400 | 12,336 | 13,264 | 10,493 |
| Prepaid closed group accrued benefits | 13,762 | 13,120 | 10,664 | 7,973 | 10,924 | 8,633 |
| Prepaid closed group accrued benefits (%) | 45.29 | 44.71 | 44.32 | 39.26 | 45.16 | 45.14 |
| Annual Cost Measures (percentages of taxable payroll) | | | | | | |
| Prepay max cost rate (%) | 18.46 | 17.77 | 14.43 | 11.04 | 14.68 | 11.59 |
| Yr of prepay max cost rate | 2035 | 2037 | 2034 | 2030 | 2037 | 2035 |
| Yr prepay cost rate less than transfer cost rate | 2054 | 2054 | 2055 | 2051 | 2053 | 2054 |
| 2080 transfer cost rate (%) | 19.51 | 18.68 | 15.86 | 9.75 | 15.57 | 12.27 |
| 2080 prepay cost rate (%) | 11.98 | 11.63 | 10.09 | 6.37 | 9.27 | 7.48 |

SOURCE: Authors' estimates.

cost rate declines with higher rates of return. This maximum is 18.5 percent in 2035 for Current Medicare when the 2.9 percent return is used, as reported in table 12-3. The lowest maximum prepayment cost rate of 11.0 percent, under the same rate-of-return assumption, is produced by 2011 Technology Medicare. Given that this reform reduces future benefits most severely, the maximum occurs earlier in 2030. At the highest rate of return, this maximum falls to 13.4 percent for Current Medicare and occurs in 2037.

The next row in the table reports the crossover year in which the prepayment costs fall below the pay-as-you-go cost-rate schedule for each

TABLE 12-4
REFORM SUMMARY MEASURES—5.2 PERCENT REAL RATE OF RETURN

| | | | | | | No-First- |
|---|---|---|---|---|---|---|
| | | Present Value Measures (in billions) | | | | |
| Summary Measure | Current | Commission | Retire Tech | 2011 Tech | Means-Test | Dollar |
| Open group unfunded | 27,769 | 26,119 | 20,645 | 14,787 | 20,089 | 14,034 |
| Closed group unfunded | 25,816 | 24,775 | 19,492 | 15,738 | 19,617 | 14,555 |
| Net open group outgo | 36,856 | 35,206 | 29,732 | 23,874 | 29,176 | 23,121 |
| Closed group accrued benefits | 30,387 | 29,346 | 24,064 | 20,309 | 24,188 | 19,126 |
| Non-prepaid closed group accrued benefits | 18,400 | 17,925 | 14,758 | 13,449 | 14,671 | 11,606 |
| Prepaid closed group accrued benefits | 11,988 | 11,421 | 9,305 | 6,860 | 9,517 | 7,520 |
| Prepaid closed group accrued benefits (%) | 39.45 | 38.92 | 38.67 | 33.78 | 39.35 | 39.32 |
| | | Annual Cost Measures (percentages of taxable payroll) | | | | |
| Prepay max cost rate (%) | 13.44 | 12.92 | 10.48 | 8.56 | 10.67 | 8.43 |
| Yr of prepay max cost rate | 2037 | 2037 | 2034 | 2030 | 2037 | 2037 |
| Yr prepay cost rate less than transfer cost rate | 2041 | 2041 | 2041 | 2038 | 2041 | 2041 |
| 2080 transfer cost rate (%) | 19.51 | 18.68 | 15.86 | 9.75 | 15.57 | 12.27 |
| 2080 prepay cost rate (%) | 5.10 | 4.90 | 4.39 | 2.79 | 3.91 | 3.17 |

SOURCE: Authors' estimates.

reform. In table 12-3, using the 2.9 percent return, the crossover year is between 2051 and 2055, depending on the reform. The 60/40 portfolio return of 5.2 percent used in table 12-4 results in crossover years of 2038–41. The final two rows allow for comparison of the pay-as-you-go cost rate to the prepaid contribution rate in 2080 for all of the reforms. The row reflecting the pay-as-you-go cost rate is the same in each table and indicates that it is higher than the prepaid rate for all of the reforms under all rate-of-return assumptions. The pay-as-you-go cost rate can also be compared to the maximum prepaid contribution rate for each reform. With the exception of 2011 Technology Medicare, the pay-as-you-go cost rate in 2080 is higher than the maximum prepaid contribution rate.

## Conclusion

This chapter outlined the techniques used to compare prepaying retirement health-care consumption for all of the reforms and for three real rate-of-return assumptions. All birth years from 1988 onward fully prepay their retirement health care, net of the premiums they will pay in retirement. Individuals who were born before 1988 and have yet to retire from the labor force also contribute to prepaying their retirement health care. They contribute at the rate that would have prepaid their retirement health care had they contributed for all of their working years. The contribution rates are determined on a cohort-by-cohort basis and are contingent on the rate of return assumed. The prepaid insurance partially offsets the benefit expected for the individuals born before 1988 and fully offsets it for individuals born in 1988 and later. The size of the benefits workers prepay is contingent on the reform we analyze.

Several conclusions can be drawn from the base comparison between prepaying Current Medicare benefits and paying for the same benefits as currently done on a pay-as-you-go basis. This comparison uses the same real rate of return in computing the prepayment contribution and cost rates as is used in producing the estimates in the *2006 Medicare Trustees Report*. First, as expected, prepayment brings the cost forward in time relative to the current arrangement. Second, the long-term prepayment contribution rate is lower than Current Medicare's cost rate with pay-as-you-go financing. Third, the long-term cohort contribution rates are neutral across generations, in that lifetime benefits are equal to lifetime contributions, while the pay-as-you-go financing arrangement has produced and will produce some cohorts who are net beneficiaries of the system and some who are net taxpayers to the system. Making the system neutral in its treatment of members of each birth year will reduce the labor-supply disincentives facing workers who expect to be net taxpayers in the current system.

The comparison of the reforms, all using the same methodology and a variety of interest rates, naturally raises the issues of judging which reform is preferred and which interest rate is the best. The reforms provide alternative ways to think about controlling Medicare's growth as a federal entitlement program. We know that the 45 percent trigger in the Medicare Modernization Act requires that discussion of Medicare reform begin in the next few years.

Only time will tell how that process will play out and how fundamental is the reform on which Congress agrees. If the enacted reform fundamentally changes the insurance structure through greater cost-sharing for all retirees, or if the greater cost-sharing is limited to higher-income retirees, the rate of growth in health-care spending will likely decline. How the other reforms are implemented will also change the rate of growth in health-care spending by retirees. But regardless of the type of reform enacted, workers will be forced to change their life-cycle consumption and saving patterns. Reduction in benefits will cause some individuals to save more during their work years if current projections approximate desired benefits.

As the results based on the different rates of return illustrate, the costs of prepaying Current Medicare or any of the reformed benefit schedules are less onerous with higher return assumptions. But even with the lower return assumption, prepayment has its advantages. The assets owned by the insurance providers determine the rate of return on the prepaid policies and will be higher than the government borrowing rate. This should approach the real gross rate of return in the economy, which is in the neighborhood of 4.7 percent. The estimated contribution rates based on the 5.2 percent rate of return are thus reasonable approximations.

We motivated the discussion of prepayment by alluding to the long-run actuarial deficit associated with Part A of Medicare. Combining all parts of Medicare, we estimated an income rate that would fund Current Medicare indefinitely and compared it to the prepayment rate through time to illustrate the potential tradeoffs. The same government borrowing rate was used to generate the respective rates, and, therefore, the two series are directly comparable. But, as we noted, partially prepaying Medicare through a single trust fund requires that the trust fund be invested in private financial assets and held independently from the federal government. Otherwise, the surplus will be spent, as the Social Security surpluses have been spent since the 1983 reforms. However, the prospect of a trust fund holding private financial-market assets of the necessary magnitude seems unlikely.

The alternative mode of prepayment through cohort-based contributions to retirement health-insurance policies must overcome the concerns associated with a single, centrally held trust fund. Thus, the insurance providers must be private. Conceptually, the prepaid insurance discussed in this and the preceding chapters is mortality-contingent, is priced at the cohort level, and pays defined real lifetime benefits similar to pensions. Private defined-benefit programs are conceptually similar; however, in recent years the prevalence of such programs has declined and is being replaced by individualized defined-contribution plans. Individualizing prepaid retirement health insurance through mandatory defined contributions to individual retirement insurance accounts is an alternative to private retirement insurance providers, but it raises other questions, namely, can the accumulated value be transferred to one's heirs? Will different birth years be treated differently by the financial markets? How will the accounts of low-income workers be subsidized to ensure sufficient funding at retirement?

Making the accounts inheritable increases the costs. As we have priced the insurance, all contributions of individuals who do not survive to retirement age are implicitly distributed to funding the health-care consumption of survivors, as is implicit in the current funding arrangement. Differential treatment of successive groups of retirees by the financial markets is a risk-taking role addressed by the private retirement insurance providers. If individualized accounts are used, then variation in returns across groups of retirees could be lessened through partial annuitization periodically during retirement, such that the annuities are sufficient to fund expected premium payments.

Redistribution would occur within cohorts by requiring contributions as a percentage of payroll. The target contribution in each year is the contribution rate times the earnings of the average cohort member. Individuals with above-average earnings would subsidize the accounts of cohort members with below-average earnings, equalizing the annual contribution amounts for all members of the cohort.

# 13

# Medicare and the Social Contract

Health-care insurance for the elderly is often referred to as a form of "social insurance." Discussions of social insurance usually comprise a handful of concepts, including the risks insurance is intended to cover, the extent of participation in the program, whether the program should be prepaid by the insurance recipients, and whether redistribution within generations and across generations is a fundamental component of such insurance. No matter the context, the idea that elderly consumption should be guaranteed through some form of social contract has a long history in the United States. In terms of health care for the general population, President Franklin D. Roosevelt, in his January 23, 1939, "Message to Congress on the National Health Program," declared,

> The objective of a national health program is to make available in all parts of our country and for all groups of our people the scientific knowledge and skill at our command to prevent and care for sickness and disability; to safeguard mothers, infants and children; and to offset through social insurance the loss of earnings among workers who are temporarily or permanently disabled (Roosevelt 1939).

Twenty-six years later, in Independence, Missouri, Lyndon B. Johnson heralded the signing of the Medicare Bill with these words:

> No longer will older Americans be denied the healing miracle of modern medicine. No longer will illness crush and destroy the savings that they have so carefully put away over a lifetime so that they might enjoy dignity in their later years. No longer

will young families see their own incomes, and their own hopes, eaten away simply because they are carrying out their deep moral obligations to their parents, and to their uncles, and their aunts. And no longer will this Nation refuse the hand of justice to those who have given a lifetime of service and wisdom and labor to the progress of this progressive country (Johnson 1965).

And at the signing of the Medicare Prescription Drug, Improvement, and Modernization Act of 2003, George W. Bush observed,

Drug coverage under Medicare will allow seniors to replace more expensive surgeries and hospitalizations with less expensive prescription medicine. And even more important, drug coverage under Medicare will save our seniors from a lot of worry. Some older Americans spend much of their Social Security checks just on their medications. Some cut down on the dosage, to make a bottle of pills last longer. Elderly Americans should not have to live with those kinds of fears and hard choices. This new law will ease the burden on seniors and will give them the extra help they need (Bush 2003).

As we come to grips with the financing issues posed by projected Medicare and impose on the system a reform that either increases the burden on the younger generation or places a significant burden on the elderly, are we abrogating a social contract? Before answering this question, let us review the concept of social insurance.

Social insurance has taken on a broad connotation. In response to the question, "What is Social Insurance?" the National Academy of Social Insurance (n.d.) offers the following statement:

Social insurance, both in the United States and abroad, encompasses broad-based systems for insuring workers and their families against economic insecurity caused by loss of income from work and the cost of health care. The Academy's work covers social insurance systems—such as Social Security, Medicare,

Workers' Compensation and unemployment insurance—and related social assistance and private employee benefits.

The bundling together of Social Security and Medicare expands the discussion of social insurance from the fundamentals of insurance to the issues of universality, transfer payments, and redistribution. But if we go back to the risks covered by each program and identify those that fall under the purview of insurance, then we can clarify the discussion and more appropriately deal with intergenerational transfers embodied in Social Security and Medicare.

Including age as an insurable risk is where "social" has to be added to "insurance." Illnesses, accidents, and spells of involuntary unemployment are all insurable risks in that they are rare and often episodic. Unemployment insurance, workers' compensation insurance, and disability insurance under Social Security are classic examples of insurance. The survivors' insurance, or life insurance, component of Social Security also falls into this category. Because of the possibility of moral hazard, it might be argued that participation in insuring against these risks should be mandatory. However, even mandatory participation does not imply that these insurance programs must be run by the government. For example, automobile liability insurance is mandatory in most states, but it is not run by state government.

Importantly, we must not let the fact that some of the risks covered by Social Security and Medicare are truly insurable risks serve as justification for the provision of the retirement consumption that forms the bulk of Social Security and Medicare expenditures. This provision can and should be separated from the insurance against random events. Because reaching the age of full Social Security and Medicare eligibility is the norm, it is not insurable. The reforms that deal with the provision of retirement consumption should be separate from any discussion of providing for the truly insurable risks. The latter are the cheaper part of any reform.

Inclusion of age as a risk that society should corporately insure may have made sense in 1935 at the inception of Social Security, when life expectancy at the age of sixty-five was about twelve years, and the probability that new entrants to the labor force in that year would reach retirement age was about 73 percent. Even then, the 73 percent chance of survival to so-called old age indicates that old age was the normal expectation. To insure against a disaster that had a 73 percent chance of occurring would be exorbitantly expensive.

Today, life expectancy for new retirees at the age of sixty-six is 18.5 years. Further, 85 percent of new entrants to the labor force will reach the 2022 full retirement age of sixty-seven, and if they reach that age, they can expect to live another 19.4 years. Reaching retirement age is thus not rare, nor is the cost of retirement random. Thus, for most people, retirement is a foreseeable event for which they can and should plan. It is conceivable that upon entry into the labor force, members of a cohort may agree to an insurance compact in which they receive benefits in retirement should they face spells of unemployment or years out of the labor force due to events beyond their control. This sort of insurance would be relatively inexpensive because few would be eligible to collect. What is important is that such insurance is inexpensive relative to the current programs, not the determination of whether it is funded by members of a specific cohort or by contemporaneous transfers.

The concept of social insurance in its broadest sense includes providing for retirement consumption through Social Security and Medicare, but these two programs should more appropriately be considered social transfers, not social insurance, because workers' tax payments are transferred to retirees not on the basis of risk, but rather on the basis of age. It is conceivable that all individuals would be expected to participate in an insurance program to compensate those who reach old age and are in poverty. All would participate in funding the insurance, but benefits would be concentrated on the few who qualify. In this way, the insurance is similar to disability insurance, survivors' insurance, workers' compensation insurance, and unemployment insurance.

Likewise, universal participation would be expected in providing for known retirement expenditures. In this case, all would participate in funding, and all would receive benefits. Some express the concern that without mandatory participation, some individuals will not save enough for retirement because they are either myopic or they underestimate the likelihood of a long life. These concerns are legitimate, and can be addressed through mandatory saving. Equity issues, often the red flag of those who advocate the current transfer-payment financing, can be easily addressed in prepaid systems through within-cohort redistribution, or can be addressed at retirement with general means-tested old-age welfare payments.

We have discussed the provision of retirement consumption primarily in terms of prepayment. This prepayment could occur through individual accounts or through contributions to pension providers. Some commentators seem to dismiss the distinction between prepayment and the current transfer-payment mechanism as being of little consequence to current and future generations. The issues related to generational equity are addressed with prepayment; more importantly, prepayment would positively affect national saving, and, as a consequence, national income.

One fact that defenders of the current program are quick to point out is that Social Security provides much of the income for most retirees, seeming to imply that without Social Security, retirees would have little or nothing on which to live. It is important that this perception be addressed. The implication that, in the absence of Social Security, retirees would not have saved is a stretch. The fact that retirees rely heavily on Social Security implies that it replaced private saving, not that the saving would not have occurred.

Redistribution within and across generations should be separate from the essential goal of providing for consumption during retirement. Prepayment of retirement consumption addresses intergenerational redistribution. Within-cohort redistribution can occur under an agreement to insure against old-age poverty. Alleviating poverty among retirees can also be accomplished with transfers from workers, but using transfers for this purpose is much less expensive than providing consumption-replacement for all retirees.

Important questions must be answered, however: Do the issues associated with the provision of retirement health-care consumption differ from those of providing for other retirement consumption? Is there more uncertainty in providing health care? Don't the facts that health risks vary from retiree to retiree and that most health-care spending is concentrated on individuals experiencing a major health shock, or who are in the last years of life, necessitate that the risks be borne by a social insurance compact?

Consider again the concept of cohort-based insurance in which new entrants to the labor force agree to finance their own retirement health care. Members of the cohort do not know who will survive to retirement or, if they survive, how long they will live and how much health care they will consume. It is conceivable that cohorts could prepay their retirement health insurance through premium payments throughout their lifetimes. Some will argue that such insurance would be too expensive for a cohort, but what they are really arguing is that a future generation should pay for the too-expensive retirees' health care. Another worry is that the cohorts will face unforeseen changes in health-care technology that may occur during their retirement years. This is a valid concern that brings up the issue of who should pay for technological advances in health care consumed by the elderly. Once individuals retire, they lose one of their best forms of insurance against economic losses—their ability to work more to compensate for them.

Given the current transfer-payment financing arrangement, it may be difficult to change the generational burdens by moving to prepayment. This is particularly true for generations that are currently living. Adjustments to Medicare and Social Security should be chosen carefully to reduce costs rather than to increase the burden borne by taxpayers. Consistent with the fundamental role of insurance, the programs should move away from their current roles as transfer programs to being insurance programs.

### Can We Retain "Social Insurance" and Reform Medicare?

There is no question that something must be done if current elderly entitlement programs are to continue.[1] In figure 13-1, we show the share of projected federal nonentitlement revenues that will be required to fund the shortfalls in Social Security and Medicare. To put the issue in perspective, consider that in 2020, covering these shortfalls will consume almost 25 percent of projected federal nonentitlement revenues. Just ten years later, in 2030, the transfers will require more than 45 percent of projected nonentitlement revenues, and, by 2040, almost 60 percent will be required to maintain these programs. Anyone looking to provide for the continuation of Social Security and Medicare must deal with this growing funding gap. It is not an illusion made up by those who favor one type of reform over another, but a real gap that must and will be dealt with by the present or some future Congress.

The Social Security and Medicare reform debate is really about how to close this funding gap—essentially, how to provide retirement benefits to current retirees as they age and to provide benefits to new retirees in the

---

1. This discussion follows the outline in Saving (2006).

very near future. How future benefits are funded, through future tax increases or through additional saving today, determines who bears the burden of closing the gap and when that burden is borne. Given that these programs must be changed, must we give up social insurance in the process?

FIGURE 13-1

SOCIAL SECURITY AND MEDICARE FUNDING SHORTFALLS AS A
PERCENTAGE OF FEDERAL NONENTITLEMENT REVENUES

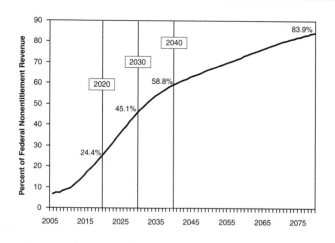

SOURCES: Authors' estimates and 2006 Social Security and Medicare Trustees Reports.
NOTE: Federal nonentitlement taxes are estimated to be 11.8 percent of GDP, the twenty-five-year average.

## Social Insurance: What Does It Mean?

The notion of "social insurance" is essentially general agreement among members of a generation that when a pitfall occurs to an individual, others will absorb all or some part of the individual's loss. Such insurance works best when the probability of a loss is low and independent across individual participants in the contract. Given this form of social insurance, should provision for retirement consumption for all individuals be part of a social contract? The probability that a member of the cohort born in 2006 will live to retirement age is 0.87. Thus, cohort members cannot insure themselves against the remote chance they will survive to retirement, since reaching retirement age is expected.

What a cohort can insure against is the likelihood that members and/or their families will suffer income losses during their work years due to premature death or disability, or that they will reach retirement age and not have sufficient resources for retirement consumption, both clear roles for social insurance. Social insurance would then have each member of the cohort placing resources in a common account and using them to compensate those unfortunate enough to have become disabled, those who have too little for retirement consumption, or the survivors of those who have died young.

Social insurance loses its meaning when one crosses generations. In fact, intergenerational social insurance is at best inefficient and at worst unworkable. Many of the current financial problems of Social Security and Medicare are the result of retired and older working cohorts pressuring Congress to give them benefits to be paid for by a combination of currently young and unborn generations, without regard for generational equity. Social Security reform is primarily about generations prepaying their retirement benefits. Such prepayment does not preclude social insurance and, in fact, provides the funds for such insurance. Thus, retirement funding reform and social insurance are not mutually exclusive.

While Social Security's problems are largely demographic in origin, Medicare's financing problem adds to the same demographic problem the fact that the demand for health care is growing faster than income. The demographic problem is a combination of decreasing fertility and mortality, both of which, in the long run, worsen the dependency ratio. Moreover, it is not the case that, even in the short run, the decrease in fertility offsets the decrease in mortality to leave the dependency ratio unchanged. In fact, the dependency ratio is rising and is expected to rise for at least the next seventy-five years.

Medicare's second problem stems from the fact that the share of total income earned in the preretirement ages that individuals choose to spend on health care is increasing. As an in-kind benefit, Medicare is a commitment to provide as much health care as retirees choose to consume. The combination of Social Security and Medicare benefits as projected by the Medicare trustees will replace a share of preretirement consumption that threatens to reach 80 percent. Assuming two workers per retiree, a level the trustees project will occur in 2040, replacing 80 percent of preretirement consumption will require each to give up 40 percent of his or her consumption. Clearly, this level of taxation is not a sustainable equilibrium.

## Conclusion

All Social Security and Medicare reforms must deal with the fact that benefits, as currently scheduled, cannot be paid with the current tax rate or, for that matter, with any conceivable tax rate. Those who favor the current financing arrangement must explicitly detail whose taxes will be raised and whose benefits will be cut. Prepayment of some or all retirement consumption, including health care, with personal retirement accounts has collateral benefits. Workers become the owners of their retirement accounts, and increased saving will increase the nation's income relative to the current financing arrangement. For these reasons, such reforms offer a promising alternative in the current policy discussion.

We must find a way for the working generation to pay for some or most of their retirement consumption while they are working. If we pay current-law benefits for Social Security and Medicare and only collect current-law taxes and premiums, the shortfalls will use up large parts of future federal nonentitlement revenues. Transfers of the magnitude necessary to pay projected benefits cannot and will not happen. The real issue is not whether, but how, these programs will be changed. It is imperative that the working population supply the resources to pay for all of their retirement consumption, including health care.

# 14

# Conclusions and Other Issues in the Medicare Reform Debate

The reform issues presented in the previous chapters have dealt with the three aspects of the Medicare program that have worked together to get us to the current situation. First, Medicare is financed through pay-as-you-go. Existing workers pay for the benefits given to the retired population—essentially a system with generational transfers as its principal source of revenue. Second, because the financing system involves generational transfers, the size of succeeding generations matters. In addition to generation size, the time spent in the workforce also matters. Third, the Medicare payment scheme ensures that users of the system will not care what it costs, implying that suppliers do not face the usual controls on prices. In this chapter, we review these and other factors that are important to the trustees' and our projections of the future of Medicare.

Given that the projections made by the trustees depend critically on assumptions concerning fertility and immigration, we will first address these issues from an international perspective. This perspective is particularly important for immigration, since the future path of U.S. immigration depends on fertility in the rest of the world and the rest of the world's demand for immigrants.

### Demographics and Medicare

Almost all discussions of Medicare's growing financing burden as a percentage of GDP point to the underlying demographics of the soon-to-retire baby boom generation and the expectation that health-care spending will outpace the growth in per-capita GDP for most of the projection period. The changing age structure of the population will occur within the next twenty-five years as those sixty-five and over, expressed as a percentage of the population of potential workers twenty to sixty-four years of age, rises from 20 percent to 35 percent. By 2080, the number of individuals in the sixty-five and older population relative to the number of individuals in the working-age population will have more than doubled from its current share to more than 42 percent. The rise in the retiree-per-worker ratio is rooted in changing fertility patterns and increasing life expectancy. This demographic effect was isolated in chapter 2 in our discussion of projected Medicare spending under the assumption that per-capita spending grows at the same rate as per-capita GDP. With that assumption, projected Medicare spending would reach 6.7 percent of GDP rather than the 11.0 percent predicted in the *2006 Medicare Trustees Report*. But the demographic effects alone more than double the size of Medicare compared to its current 3.21 percent of GDP.

The population age structures in other large economies are predicted to undergo rapid changes over the next twenty-five years as well. In fact, relative to the other G8 countries, forecasts by both the United Nations and the U.S. Census Bureau predict that the percentage of the population sixty-five years of age and over in the United States will be much smaller in the long run than in other parts of the developed world. The Census Bureau (2006) estimates that in 2030, 19.6 percent of the population in the United States will be sixty-five or over. While this increase in the share of elderly in the U.S. population is significant, in Japan and Germany, for example, the proportion is expected to be 28 percent and 27 percent, respectively. Further, for these latter two countries, the Census Bureau's fertility-rate projections for 2030 are only 1.56, compared to the trustees' projection for the United States of a long-run fertility rate of 2.00. Thus, the elderly population share in other developed countries is projected to continue to rise faster than our own.

In spite of a fertility rate below that required to sustain the U.S. population, the trustees forecast that it will continue to grow by 41 percent over the seventy-five-year projection period. Given the ultimate fertility rate of 2.00—just below the 2.05 fertility rate of the last decade and below the population-sustaining rate of 2.10—the population growth projected by the trustees is due entirely to immigration. Given that the entire developed world will have an increasing need for immigrants as we move further into the twenty-first century, the assumption that the United States will receive the level of immigration required to meet the population projections of the trustees is open to serious question. The question is, then, with fertility declining in even the growing nations, will the demand for immigrants increase their value enough to make the trustees' assumptions too optimistic?[1] Only time will tell.

While demographic considerations are a key part of understanding Medicare's funding predicament, when we go back to our analysis in chapters 5–8, which assumed that the underlying demographics are the same across all reforms, we are left with growing federal budget pressures regardless of the reform in question. Those pressures result from the current generational-transfer financing nature of these programs. Moving to prepayment can alleviate some of the generational inequities we have seen.

## The Magnitude of the Problem

In chapters 3 and 4, we estimated the impact of Medicare's future funding shortfalls on the nation by assuming that the non-Medicare entitlement role of the federal government in the economy would remain at its 2006 level. Under this condition, we calculated the increase in taxation that would be required to fund Current Medicare. Expressed in terms of payroll, and assuming that we leave the federal government non-Medicare entitlement spending at its current share of GDP, the tax rate required by the close of the trustees' seventy-five-year projection period to fund Medicare is virtually 20 percent, almost seven times the current 2.9 percent Medicare payroll tax rate.[2]

Alternatively, under the assumption that we require the elderly to make up the deficits, we estimated that the premiums needed for Medicare Part

---

1. The United Nations estimates that by 2050, fertility in the G8 countries plus India and China will be 1.80 (United Nations 2004).

2. Leaving the non-Medicare federal entitlement spending at its current share of GDP implies a decreasing size of government over time, as both Social Security and Medicaid will consume ever-larger shares of revenues.

B would rise rapidly from their current level of 25 percent of expenditures to 42 percent of expenditures in 2020, 57 percent in 2030, and 65 percent in 2040. The Medicare Part D numbers are even more startling. Part D premiums would have to increase from their current level of roughly 22.8 percent of expenditures to 67 percent in just fifteen years—by 2020—and then to 78 percent by 2030 and 81 percent by 2040. Finally, at the close of the seventy-five-year projection period, the Part B premium would have to account for more than 74 percent of total Part B expenditures, and the Part D premium for 86 percent of total Part D expenditures.

While the numbers for Parts B and D are eye-opening, when we add the Medicare Part A premiums to them, they become staggering. If we used premiums rather than payroll taxation to pay for the projected Part A deficits, Part A premiums would rise from their current zero level to 24 percent of total Part A expenditures by 2020, 44 percent by 2030, and 56 percent by 2040. Finally, at the close of the trustees' seventy-five-year projection period, Part A premiums would have to account for more than 70 percent of total Part A expenditures.

Premiums at the levels required to keep the Medicare transfer at its current share of federal nonentitlement revenues would place a significant burden on the elderly. One way of measuring its extent is to express the premiums as a percentage of projected Social Security benefits. The projected premiums would exhaust most and, for some higher-earners, all of projected Social Security benefits by the close of the seventy-five-year projection period. For scaled high-earners, the premiums would require more than 78 percent of Social Security benefits, leaving less than 22 percent for consumption. For scaled medium-earners, the projection is even bleaker. The premiums we project would use up all of a medium-earner's benefit. At these levels, unless all the aged were required to be part of Medicare, massive pullouts would be expected as the healthy leave, putting Medicare into a death spiral.

### What Are We Getting for Our Money?

There is considerable evidence that the expansion in expenditures on health care over the last four decades has led to increased life expectancy and improved quality of life. On the other side, however, is the evidence that very significant reductions in the level of spending have little or no effect on health status when the reductions result from higher cost-sharing. For example, in the RAND Health Insurance Experiment that we utilized for our estimates of the impact of the no-first-dollar reform scored in chapter 7, the reductions in expenditures realized by the group participating in the highest deductible policy relative to those in the free-care plan was almost 50 percent for outpatient and more than 25 percent for hospital expenditures. Importantly, there was no significant difference in the health outcomes of those participating in the cost-sharing plans and the Health Maintenance Organizations and those participating in the free-care plan (Newhouse 1993).

While the overall level of health may not be affected by a considerable reduction in health-care spending, it may still be the case that the larger-than-necessary levels of Medicare expenditures are worth the money. For example, David Cutler (1999) argues that if we assume that all of the improvements in elderly morbidity and mortality are attributable to Medicare expenditures, then these expenditures were a good investment. That is not to say, however, that we could not have achieved the same result with much less spending. In fact, in the same study, Cutler shows some evidence indicating that as much as one-third of medical care is either inappropriate or of questionable value.

Using data from the RAND study to form a basis for evaluating Medicare reform raises an important issue. The RAND study population consists of working-age individuals and may not apply fully to the elderly Medicare population. Further evidence on this point is contained in Wennberg et al. (2005) of the Dartmouth Atlas of Health Care Project. Wennberg et al. find that, based on Medicare data from California providers of care to the chronically ill, "greater spending, more resource inputs, and more frequent use of hospitals and physician services are not associated with better performance on technical measures of the processes of care."

The important question for Medicare reform, however, is whether giving the consumers a greater financial stake in their choice of care will adversely affect the general health status of the elderly. We know from the perspective of the working population that considerable by-choice reductions in health-care spending did not affect their overall health, suggesting that individuals are able to determine when consumption through health-care providers is necessary. There is no reason to believe that for the majority of the elderly the same is not true. For our purposes, however, we leave this important question for further work.

## How Far Can Reform Take Us?

The purpose of this exercise was to show that the magnitude of the Medicare problem is such that reform is necessary. But what does reform buy? In spite of the number of suggested reforms, actual accountings of their benefits are rare. In this work, we evaluated five reforms in terms of their impacts on the transfers necessary to pay for Medicare, as projected by the Medicare trustees. All reforms have one thing in common: They reduce the level of benefits received by the elderly and transfer some of the burden of paying for Medicare from taxpayers to beneficiaries.

The most surprising thing coming from the evaluation is how little the reforms accomplish or, more importantly, how large the problem is based on current projections. A partial explanation of the inability of reform to solve Medicare's financial crisis is the fact that the demand for health care is growing so much faster than the nation's output. Thus, individuals left to their own devices, and faced with the incentive inherent in the current payment environment, are opting to spend a greater and greater share of their income on those things we have categorized as health care. Unless a reform can alter this fundamental fact of life—which the No-First-Dollar Medicare reform does to some extent—it cannot have a major impact on the program's financial future.

Since the various reforms all involve some benefit reduction, if the elderly still desire to consume the level of health care underlying the trustees' projections, they will have to provide the missing funding. In effect, all reforms result in some level of prepayment, albeit informal prepayment, as workers prepare for a retirement during which they must pay for a greater share of their health care. Retirees facing higher relative prices through greater cost-sharing will reduce their consumption of health care, and the current projected spending on health care will likely overestimate the realized spending.

The transition inherent in the prepaying schedules discussed in chapters 11 and 12 requires initial contributions from workers that are in excess of currently existing tax rates, but future taxes that are much lower than those that would exist if currently scheduled Medicare benefits were paid with contemporaneous taxes. Thus, the transition does not necessarily make the early participants in the system better off, although the later generations that participate after the debts are paid in full are clearly better off. Future generations will be better off as a result of the larger capital stock they will inherit; however, the current generation must give up current consumption to generate this larger capital stock.[3]

Once a payment mechanism is put into place, the youngest members of the labor force will be setting aside the full amount for their future reformed Medicare. For them and all who follow, there will be no required general-revenue transfers and thus no unfunded liability. No matter which reform is chosen, however, the closed-group liability at the time of the reform will still exist. It is this liability that must be paid during the transition to fully prepaid Medicare. Each of the reforms analyzed erased some of the seventy-five-year unfunded liability. Figure 14-1 shows the percentage of the $30.2 trillion liability projected by the 2006 Medicare Trustees Report that would be eliminated by each of the five reforms.

The debt reduction shown in figure 14-1 applies to the open-group Medicare debt, meaning that seventy-five new cohorts enter the system over the calculation period. When full prepayment is introduced, cohorts entering the system after its introduction impose no unfunded debt on the system, but must pay taxes in addition to contributing to the prepayment of Medicare. Therefore, the open-group debt is not the measure of the amount of debt that must be covered by current and future workers. Rather, it is the reformed closed-group debt that must be paid through additional taxation during the transition to fully prepaid Medicare.

The closed-group unfunded liability for Current Medicare from the 2006 Medicare Trustees Report is $27.9 trillion. The effect of a reform on this

---

3. See Feldstein and Samwick (1997) for a discussion of the possibility of a Pareto improving transition in the context of prefunding Social Security and Medicare benefits. Also see Kotlikoff (1995) for another discussion of efficiency gains resulting from prepaying Social Security and tax reform.

FIGURE 14-1
PERCENTAGE OF CURRENT MEDICARE'S SEVENTY-FIVE-YEAR
UNFUNDED LIABILITY PAID OFF: ALL REFORMS

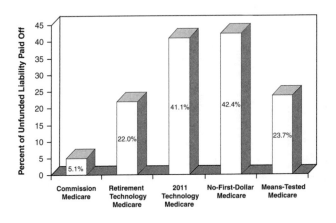

SOURCE: Authors' estimates.
NOTE: Restricted to beneficiaries 65 and older.

amount depends on how it treats existing retirees. Only one of the five reforms analyzed fails to affect current retirees. Commission Medicare extends the number of years existing nonretirees must live before becoming eligible for Medicare, but does not take away benefits from anyone receiving Medicare at the time the reform is instituted. The remaining reforms treat those already retired at the time of implementation in the same fashion as new retirees. No-First-Dollar Medicare is applied to all current and future retirees, as is Means-Tested Medicare. Both Retirement Technology Medicare and 2011 Technology Medicare apply to those retiring beginning in 2011, and both impose the 2011 profile on all beneficiaries of Medicare in 2011.

In chapter 12 we reported the closed-group debt for Current Medicare and all five reforms. The closed-group debt is important because after the prepayment reform is introduced, all new entrants to the labor force will be fully prepaying their future Medicare expenses. Thus, the closed-group debt must be paid through taxation and during the lifetimes of all those in the closed group. In figure 14-2, we show the closed-group unfunded liability for Current Medicare and the five reforms. When prepayment is in its long-run equilibrium, the closed-group unfunded liability must be totally paid off. The burden imposed on new entrants depends on which reform, if any, is chosen, and on how the prepayment is instituted.

FIGURE 14-2
CLOSED-GROUP UNFUNDED LIABILITY

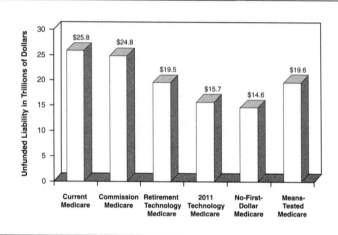

SOURCE: Authors' estimates.
NOTE: Restricted to beneficiaries 65 and older.

The prepayment rule we set out in chapter 11 imposes a constant work-life contribution rate as a percentage of payroll that would prepay each cohort's projected health-care expenditures, for all existing and future cohorts. Thus, all new cohorts totally prepay their retirement health care. Further, all cohorts in the closed group will contribute toward their retirement health-care expenditures but will not totally prepay them. Because members of the closed group are making contributions toward, but not totally prepaying, their retirement health-care benefits, the closed-group unfunded liability reported in figure 14-2 will be reduced by the contributions made by members of the closed group.

The after-prepayment closed-group unfunded liability is affected by the real rate of return assumed, since this real rate affects the estimated contribution rates. Because the contribution rates are set to achieve a balance at age sixty-five equal to the age sixty-five value of projected healthcare expenditures for each cohort, they are inversely related to the real rate of return assumed. The greater the rate of return underlying the contribution rates, the lower the required contribution rate. As a result, the post-prepayment closed-group unfunded obligation is inversely related to the assumed real rate of return.

In figure 14-3 we show the post-prepayment closed-group unfunded obligation for the government-borrowing real rate of return of 2.9 percent. For Current Medicare and all reforms, the introduction of prepayment in the manner we described in chapter 11 reduces the closed-group unfunded liability by about 45 percent, with one exception—2011 Technology Medicare—where the reduction is only 40 percent.

FIGURE 14-3
**AFTER PREPAYMENT CLOSED-GROUP UNFUNDED LIABILITY**
**2.9 Percent Real Rate of Return**

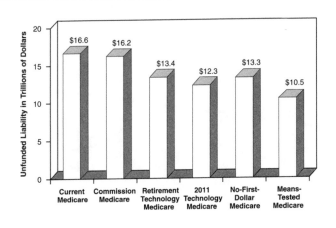

SOURCE: Authors' estimates.
NOTE: Restricted to beneficiaries 65 and older.

The important point here is that even after the introduction of a prepayment mechanism that requires all working members of the closed group to make contributions toward their future retirement health-care consumption, there still remains a significant closed-group unfunded liability that must be paid with taxation. Because the term of the closed group is one hundred years, the taxation must all occur in that period of time.

As an example of the level of taxation implied by the introduction of a prepayment system, we show the tax rates required to pay off the post-prepayment closed-group debt for Current Medicare in figure 14-4.[4] These are tax rates that apply to the open group in that all workers pay the taxes. At its introduction in 2006, the tax rate was 4.86 percent, just under two percentage points above the current 2.9 percent HI tax rate. The tax rate peaks in 2032 at 7.93 percent and then falls. The transition tax rate finally falls below the current HI tax rate in 2057 and reaches zero in 2088.

FIGURE 14-4

OPEN-GROUP TAX RATE REQUIRED TO PAY OFF CURRENT
MEDICARE POST-PREPAYMENT CLOSED-GROUP DEBT

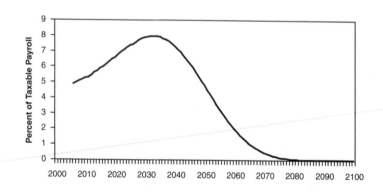

SOURCE: Authors' estimates.
NOTE: Non-prepaid closed group costs are calculated assuming prepaid retirement insurance earns a rate of return equal to the government borrowing rate.

---

4. For an expanded discussion of the issues of the transition from a pay-as-you-go elderly entitlement system to a prepaid system, see Liu, Rettenmaier, and Saving (2005).

In our analysis we derived the contribution rates that would have allowed each birth cohort to prepay its retirement medical expenditures had its members contributed in each year they were in the labor force. These contribution rates imply a lifetime contribution rate that is considerably less than the lifetime tax rate that would be required for Current Medicare. Even with a very conservative assumption concerning the rate of return—the real government rate of 2.9 percent assumed by the Medicare trustees—all those born after 1980 could have prepaid Medicare with lifetime contribution rates that are less than the lifetime tax rates they will face if Current Medicare continues. At a still conservative, but higher, real rate of return of 5.2 percent, all those born after 1941, including all of the baby boomers, could have prepaid Medicare with lifetime contribution rates that are less than the lifetime tax rates they have faced and will face with Current Medicare. As we have discussed, the fact that most Medicare revenues come from taxpayers rather than retirees will continually place the program on the public policy hot seat. Full prepayment, as we have outlined, will move Medicare off the public policy agenda, and even partial prepayment will make it less politically charged.

## Conclusion

In the end, our diagnosis of Medicare's ailments has identified a couple of persisting conditions. The first is a financing mechanism built on transfers from taxpayers to retirees. The continuation of Medicare as currently structured implies ever-growing burdens on future taxpayers. This arrangement also separates the consumers of health care from the people who are paying the bills. As a result, the program's financing is a political issue that places one group in opposition to another. To the extent that members of Congress are aided by the complexity of Medicare and their ability to micromanage the current system, they lose power by allowing individuals to be in control of their own Medicare accounts. Further, the arrangement has produced a situation in which early beneficiaries have received and continue to receive significantly higher benefits than are warranted by their lifetime taxes in support of the program. The benefits to the early participants come at the expense of all future generations in the form of a reduced level of national investment and lower potential income than would exist if flows from workers' accumulated savings rather than transfers from taxpayers had to fund their retirements.

Medicare's other persisting condition is the current cost-sharing arrangement that has, in many respects, made the program a first-dollar coverage insurance policy with the presence of Medigap insurance and Medicaid coverage. Throughout their working years, most current retirees and their dependents were covered by employer-based insurance, given that premium payments through the employer were not taxed. By the time workers reach retirement, they expect the same sort of arrangement and access to care that they had while working. But the preferential tax treatment reduces the cost of health care relative to other products and services and leads to higher consumption than would exist if the tax treatment were the same. The low amounts of cost-sharing on the part of consumers, both young and old, creates a market in which consumers and providers have limited incentives to be concerned about health-care costs, and both the level of health-care consumption and the growth rate of that consumption are affected.

The diagnosis leads to the inevitable conclusion that the program will be reformed, and that fundamental reform is necessary to address the magnitude of the projected spending. We examined a handful of treatments for these conditions. The initial treatments we considered primarily constrain Medicare's costs as paid for by taxpayers. Reducing taxpayers' financial commitment to the program can be achieved by raising the retirement age, constraining the growth in the transfers by making retirees responsible for financing excess cost-growth during their retirement years, means-testing the transfers so that high-income retirees receive lower transfers, and increasing the level of cost-sharing on the part of retirees. Each reform by itself would affect the generational burden, would implicitly produce partial prepayment given that current workers would be responsible for a greater share of their retirement health-care consumption, and would affect the ultimate level of and growth rate in health-care consumption.

We also examined a treatment that could be combined with any of the cost-saving reforms: prepaying retirement health-care spending rather than relying on the current transfer-payment arrangement. Such a move would be a fundamental change to the way the system is financed but, if combined with a reform of Medicare's insurance coverage that includes greater cost-sharing, would ultimately address long-run generational equity. It would also lead to a health-care market that is directed more by consumer choices and less by other means of allocating the level and quantity of care consumers receive. Ultimately, Medicare reform should be guided by the goals of achieving a more equitable distribution of burdens across generations and a more economically efficient mix of health-care and non-health-care consumption.

# References

Auerbach, Alan J., Laurence J. Kotlikoff, and Willi Leibfritz (eds.). 1999. *General Accounting around the World*. Chicago: University of Chicago Press.

Bell, Felicitie C., and Michael L. Miller. 2005. *Life Tables for the United States Social Security Area 1900-2100*. Actuarial Study No. 120, SSA Pub. No. 11-11536 Social Security Administration, Office of the Chief Actuary, Baltimore, Md. Available at: http://www.ssa.gov/OACT/NOTES/s2000s.html, accessed on February 19, 2007.

The Board of Trustees, Federal Hospital Insurance and Federal Supplementary Medical Insurance Trust Funds. 2006. *The Annual Report of the Boards of Trustees of the Federal Hospital Insurance and Federal Supplementary Medical Insurance Trust Funds*. Washington, D.C.: U.S. Government Printing Office.

The Board of Trustees, Federal Old-Age and Survivors Insurance and Federal Disability Insurance Trust Funds. 2006. *The 2006 Annual Report of the Board of Trustees of the Federal Old-Age and Survivors Insurance and Federal Disability Insurance Trust Funds*. Washington, D.C.: U.S. Government Printing Office.

Bush, George W. 2003. President Signs Medicare Legislation: Remarks by the President at Signing of the Medicare Prescription Drug Improvement and Modernization Act of 2003, December 8. In *Presidential Statements: George W. Bush—2003*. Social Security Online. http://www.ssa.gov/history/gwbushstmts3.html#12082003 (accessed February 14, 2007).

Christensen, Sandra, and Judy Shinogle. 1997. Effects of Supplemental Coverage on Use of Services by Medicare Enrollees. *Health Care Financing Review* 19 (1): 5–17.

Cutler, David M., 1999. What Does Medicare Spending Buy Us? In *Medicare Reform: Issues and Answers*. Bush School Series in Economics of Public Policy, vol. 1. Chicago: University of Chicago Press.

Feldstein, Martin S., and Andrew J. Samwick. 1997. The Economics of Prefunding Social Security and Medicare Benefits. National Bureau of Economic Research. Working Paper 6055. June 1997.

Frech, H. E. III. 1999. The Forgotten Opportunity of Reforming Fee-for-Service Medicare. In *Medicare in the Twenty-First Century*, ed. Robert B. Helms. Washington, D.C.: AEI Press.

Gramm, Phil, Andrew J. Rettenmaier, and Thomas R. Saving. 1998. Medicare Policy for Future Generations. *New England Journal of Medicine* 338 (April 30): 1307–10.

Johnson, Lyndon B. 1965. Remarks with President Truman at the Signing in Independence of the Medicare Bill, July 30. In *Presidential Statements: Lyndon B. Johnson.* Social Security Online. http://www.ssa.gov/history/lbjstmts.html#medicare (accessed February 14, 2007).

Kotlikoff, Laurence. 1995. *Privatization of Social Security: How it Works and Why it Matters.* Institute for Economic Development. Discussion Paper Series, No. 66. October.

Kotlikoff, Laurence, and Scott Burns. 2003. *The Coming Generational Storm.* Cambridge, Mass.: MIT Press.

Liu, Liqun, Andrew J. Rettenmaier, and Thomas R. Saving. 2005. Discounting According to Output Type. *Southern Economic Journal* 72 (1): 213–23.

Manning, Willard G., Joseph Newhouse, Naihua Duan, Emmett Keeler, Bernadette Benjamin, Arleen Leibowitz, M. Susan Marquis, and Jack Zwanziger. 1988. *Health Insurance and the Demand for Medical Care: Evidence from a Randomized Experiment.* RAND Corporation. http://www.rand.org/pubs/reports/2005/R3476.pdf (accessed February 14, 2007).

National Academy of Social Insurance. n.d. Q & A's on the National Academy of Social Insurance. http://www.nasi.org/info-url_nocat2708/info-url_nocat_show.htm?doc_id=50066 (accessed February 14, 2007).

National Bipartisan Commission on the Future of Medicare. 1999. *Final Breaux-Thomas Medicare Reform Proposal,* by John Breaux and Bill Thomas. March 1999. http://medicare.commission.gov/medicare/bbmtt31599.html (accessed February 14, 2007).

Newhouse, Joseph P. 1993. *Free for All?* Cambridge, Mass.: Harvard University Press.

Pauly, Mark V. 1999a. Can Beneficiaries Save Medicare? In *Medicare in the Twenty-First Century,* ed. Robert B. Helms. Washington, D.C.: AEI Press.

———. 1999b. Should Medicare Be Less Generous to Higher-Income Beneficiaries? In *Medicare Reform: Issues and Answers.* Bush School Series in Economics of Public Policy, vol. 1. Chicago: University of Chicago Press.

Phelps, Charles E. 1997. *Health Economics.* 2d ed. Reading, Mass.: Addison-Wesley.

Rettenmaier, Andrew J., and Thomas R. Saving. 2000. *The Economics of Medicare Reform.* Kalamazoo, Mich.: W. E. Upjohn Institute for Employment Research.

Roosevelt, Franklin D. 1939. Message to Congress on the National Health Program, January 23. In *Presidential Statements: FDR's Statements on Social Security.* Social Security Online. http://www.ssa.gov/history/fdrstmts.html#12 (accessed February 14, 2007).

———. 1944. State of the Union Message to Congress. Speech presented to Congress, Washington, D.C., January 11, 1944. http://www.presidency.ucsb.edu/ws/?pid=16518

Saving, Thomas R. 2006. Social Insurance and Elderly Entitlement Reform: Are They Compatible? *Health Affairs,* March 21, 2006.

Shaviro, Daniel. 2004. *Who Should Pay for Medicare?* Chicago: University of Chicago Press.

Sheils, John, and Randall Haught. 2004. The Cost of Tax-Exempt Health Benefits in 2004. *Health Affairs Web Exclusive* W4, February. http://content.healthaffairs.org/webexclusives/index.dtl?year=2004 (accessed February 12, 2007).

Thomasson, Melissa. 2003. The Importance of Group Coverage: How Tax Policy Shaped U.S. Health Insurance. *American Economic Review* 93 (4): 1373–84.

U.S. Census Bureau. 2006. International Data Base. http://www.census.gov/cgi-bin/ipc/idbagg (accessed February 12, 2007).

U.S. Department of Health and Human Services. Centers for Medicare and Medicaid Services. Medicare Current Beneficiary Survey (MCBS). http://www.cms.hhs.gov/LimitedDataSets/11_MCBS.asp#TopOfPage (accessed February 14, 2007).

U.S. Department of Health and Human Services. Centers for Medicare and Medicaid Services. Office of Information Services. 2004. Continuous Medicare History Sample (CMHS).

U.S. Department of Health and Human Services. Centers for Medicare and Medicaid Services. Office of the Actuary. 2006. 2006 *Annual Report of the Boards of Trustees of the Federal Hospital Insurance and Federal Supplementary Medical Insurance Trust Funds.* http://www.cms.hhs.gov/ReportsTrustFunds/downloads/tr2006.pdf (accessed February 14, 2007).

U.S. Department of Health and Human Services. National Center for Health Statistics. 1994. National Health Interview Survey (NHIS). http://www.cdc.gov/nchs/about/major/nhis/quest_data_related_1969_96a.htm#1994_NHIS (accessed February 14, 2007).

U.S. Federal Reserve Board. 2004. Survey of Consumer Finances (SCF). http://www.federalreserve.gov/pubs/oss/oss2/2004/scf2004home.html (accessed February 14, 2007).

U.S. Social Security Administration. Office of the Chief Actuary. 2005. *Scaled Factors for Hypothetical Earnings Examples Under the 2005 Trustees Report Assumptions*, by Michael Clingman and Orlo Nichols. Actuarial Note No. 2005.3.

U.S. Social Security Administration, Office of Policy. 2006. *Annual Statistical Supplement to the Social Security Bulletin, 2005*, SSA Publication No. 13-11700, February 2006.

United Nations. Department of Economic and Social Affairs. Population Division. 2004. *World Population Prospects: The 2004 Revision and World Urbanization Prospects.* http://esa.un.org/unpp/p2k0data.asp (accessed February 12, 2007).

Wennberg, John E., Elliott S. Fisher, Laurence Baker, Sandra M. Sharp, and Kristen K. Bronner. 2005. Evaluating The Efficiency of California Providers in Caring for Patients With Chronic Illnesses. *Health Affairs Web Exclusive* W5. November, 526–43. http://content.healthaffairs.org/webexclusives/index.dtl?year=2005 (accessed February 12, 2007).

# About the Authors

**Andrew J. Rettenmaier** is the executive associate director at the Private Enterprise Research Center at Texas A&M University. He received a B.B.A. in finance and a Ph.D. in economics from Texas A&M University. He is an adjunct associate professor at Texas A&M University and a senior fellow at the National Center for Policy Analysis. His primary areas of research are labor and public policy economics. Dr. Rettenmaier has co-authored with Thomas R. Saving a previous book on Medicare, *The Economics of Medicare Reform* (W. E. Upjohn Institute, 2000). They are also editors of *Medicare Reform: Issues and Answers* (University of Chicago Press, 1999).

**Thomas R. Saving** is director of the Private Enterprise Research Center at Texas A&M University. A university distinguished professor of economics at Texas A&M University, he also holds the Jeff Montgomery professorship in economics and is a senior fellow at the National Center for Policy Analysis. Dr. Saving received his Ph.D. from the University of Chicago and served on the faculty at the University of Washington at Seattle and Michigan State University before moving to Texas A&M University in 1968. He is currently co-editor of *Economic Inquiry*. His current research emphasis is on the benefit of markets in solving the pressing issues in health care and Social Security. He is the co-editor of *Medicare Reform: Issues and Answers* (University of Chicago Press, 1999), and the co-author of *The Economics of Medicare Reform* (W. E. Upjohn Institute, 2000). Dr. Saving has been president of the Western Economics Association, the Southern Economics Association, and the Association of Private Enterprise Education. In 2000, President Clinton appointed Dr. Saving as a public trustee of the Social Security and Medicare Trust Funds. On May 2, 2001, President Bush named Dr. Saving to the bipartisan President's Commission

171

to Strengthen Social Security. On April 19, 2006, President Bush appointed Dr. Saving for a second term as a public trustee of the Social Security and Medicare Trust Funds.

# Index